Headache in Otolaryngology: Rhinogenic and Beyond

Editors

HOWARD LEVINE
MICHAEL SETZEN

OTOLARYNGOLOGIC CLINICS OF NORTH AMERICA

www.oto.theclinics.com

April 2014 • Volume 47 • Number 2

ELSEVIER

1600 John F. Kennedy Boulevard • Suite 1800 • Philadelphia, Pennsylvania, 19103-2899

http://www.oto.theclinics.com

OTOLARYNGOLOGIC CLINICS OF NORTH AMERICA Volume 47, Number 2
April 2014 ISSN 0030-6665, ISBN-13: 978-0-323-29006-7

Editor: Joanne Husovski
Developmental Editor: Susan Showalter

Otolaryngologic Clinics of North America (ISSN 0030-6665) is published bimonthly by Elsevier, Inc., 360 Park Avenue South, New York, NY 10010-1710. Months of issue are February, April, June, August, October, and December. Business and Editorial Offices: 1600 John F. Kennedy Blvd., Suite 1800, Philadelphia, PA 19103-2899. Customer Service Office: 6277 Sea Harbor Drive, Orlando, FL 32887-4800. Periodicals postage paid at New York, NY and additional mailing offices. Subscription prices are $365.00 per year (US individuals), $692.00 per year (US institutions), $175.00 per year (US student/resident), $485.00 per year (Canadian individuals), $876.00 per year (Canadian institutions), $540.00 per year (international individuals), $876.00 per year (international institutions), $270.00 per year (international & Canadian student/resident). Foreign air speed delivery is included in all *Clinics'* subscription prices. All prices are subject to change without notice. **POSTMASTER:** Send address changes to *Otolaryngologic Clinics of North America*, Elsevier Health Sciences Division, Subscription Customer Service, 3251 Riverport Lane, Maryland Heights, MO 63043. **Telephone: 1-800-654-2452 (U.S. and Canada); 314-447-8871 (outside U.S. and Canada). Fax: 314-447-8029. E-mail: journalscustomerservice-usa@elsevier.com (for print support); journalsonlinesupport-usa@elsevier.com (for online support).**

Reprints. For copies of 100 or more of articles in this publication, please contact the Commercial Reprints Department, Elsevier Inc., 360 Park Avenue South, New York, NY 10010-1710. Tel.: 212-633-3874; Fax: 212-633-3820; E-mail: reprints@elsevier.com.

Otolaryngologic Clinics of North America is also published in Spanish by McGraw-Hill Interamericana Editores S.A., P.O. Box 5-237, 06500 Mexico D.F., Mexico.

Otolaryngologic Clinics of North America is covered in *MEDLINE/PubMed (Index Medicus), Current Contents/Clinical Medicine, Excerpta Medica, BIOSIS, Science Citation Index,* and *ISI/BIOMED.*

Contributors

EDITORS

HOWARD LEVINE, MD, FACS, FARS
Associate Staff, Head and Neck Institute, The Cleveland Clinic, VP Medical Affairs, Acclarent, Inc, Menlo Park, California

MICHAEL SETZEN, MD, FACS, FAAP
Clinical Associate Professor, Department of Otolaryngology, New York University Langone School of Medicine; Section Chief Rhinology, North Shore University Hospital at Manhasset, New York

AUTHORS

ALIYE BRICKER, MD
Associate Staff, Division of Neuroradiology, Cleveland Clinic Foundation, Cleveland, Ohio

JEFFREY A. BROWN, MD, FAANS, FACS
Neurological Surgery, PC, Great Neck, New York

ROGER K. CADY, MD
Headache Care Center, Springfield, Missouri

SUJANA S. CHANDRASEKHAR, MD, FACS
Director, New York Otology, New York; Director of Neurotology, James J. Peters Veterans Administration Medical Center, Bronx; Director of Neurotology, New York Head and Neck Institute, Northshore-LIJ Medical Center, New York; Clinical Associate Professor of Otolaryngology, Mount Sinai School of Medicine, New York, New York

LAURA J. DAVILA, DDS
Chief Resident, General Practice, Division of Dentistry and Oral & Maxillofacial Surgery, Weill-Cornell Medical College, New York Presbyterian Hospital, Cornell University, New York, New York

JOHN M. DELGAUDIO, MD
Department of Otolaryngology/Head and Neck Surgery, Emory University School of Medicine, Atlanta, Georgia

MERLE DIAMOND, MD
Diamond Headache Clinic, Chicago, Illinois

ALEXANDER FEOKTISTOV, MD, PhD
Diamond Headache Clinic, Chicago, Illinois

FREDERICK G. FREITAG, DO, FAHS
Associate Professor, Department of Neurology, Medical College of Wisconsin, Milwaukee, Wisconsin

CHANTAL HOLY, PhD
Director, Health Economics and Value Proposition, Acclarent, Inc, Menlo Park, California

MOHAMMAD NADIR IJAZ
Houston, Texas

HOWARD A. ISRAEL, DDS
Professor of Clinical Surgery, Division of Dentistry and Oral & Maxillofacial Surgery, Weill-Cornell Medical College, New York Presbyterian Hospital, Cornell University; Adjunct Professor of Clinical Dentistry, Columbia University College of Dental Medicine, New York, New York

DARA G. JAMIESON, MD
Associate Professor of Clinical Neurology, Weill Cornell Medical College, New York Presbyterian Hospital, New York

HOWARD LEVINE, MD, FACS, FARS
Associate Staff, Head and Neck Institute, The Cleveland Clinic, VP Medical Affairs, Acclarent, Inc, Menlo Park, California

MARK E. MEHLE, MD, FACS
Assistant Clinical Professor, Northeast Ohio Medical University, Ohio; Private Practice, ENT and Allergy Health Services, Cleveland, Ohio

RAZA PASHA, MD
Pasha Snoring and Sinus Center, Houston, Texas

ZARA M. PATEL, MD
Department of Otolaryngology/Head and Neck Surgery, Emory University School of Medicine, Atlanta, Georgia

DAVID M. POETKER, MD
Division of Otolaryngology, Department of Surgery, Zablocki VAMC, Milwaukee, Wisconsin

FALLON SCHLOEMER, DO
Department of Neurology, Froedtert Hospital, Medical College of Wisconsin, Milwaukee, Wisconsin

CURTIS P. SCHREIBER, MD
Neurologist and Headache Specialist in Private Practice, Citizens Memorial Healthcare, Bolivar, Missouri

MICHAEL SETZEN, MD, FACS, FAAP
Clinical Associate Professor, Department of Otolaryngology, New York University Langone School of Medicine; Section Chief Rhinology, North Shore University Hospital at Manhasset, New York

RAFAY QAMER SOLEJA
University of Texas Medical Branch, League City, Texas

TODD STULTZ, MD, DDS
Staff, Division of Neuroradiology, Cleveland Clinic Foundation, Cleveland, Ohio

Contents

orbital involvement, and more aggressive infectious and neoplastic processes.

We review the therapies for primary headache disorders: migraine, chronic migraine, tension-type headache, and cluster headache. Recommendations follow the evidence-based treatments so far as is possible with expert opinion to give clinical guidance. Headache has 2 levels of care: acute treatments designed to stop a headache from progressing and alleviate all symptoms associated with the headache and preventive therapies for patients whose headache frequency is such that by itself produces significant disability and impact on quality of life, or where the frequency of use of acute medications, regardless of efficacy, poses risks in terms of overuse or adverse events.

Nonneurologists who treat patients with headaches should be able recognize common headache types and to initiate therapy for tension-type headaches and migraines. Patients with complicated headache scenarios should be referred to a neurologist for consultation.

Sinus headache is a common presenting complaint in the otolaryngology office. Although most patients with this presentation are found to have migraine headache, many do not, and others fail therapy. This review focuses on the current understanding of nonneoplastic rhinogenic headache: headaches that are caused or exacerbated by nasal or paranasal sinus disease or anatomy. The literature regarding this topic is reviewed, along with a review of surgical series seeking to correct these abnormalities and the outcomes obtained with intervention. Suggestions are provided regarding patient diagnosis and management, and options for intervention are reviewed.

Patients, primary care doctors, neurologists and otolaryngologists often have differing views on what is truly causing headache in the sinonasal region. This review discusses common primary headache diagnoses that can masquerade as "sinus headache" or "rhinogenic headache," such as migraine, trigeminal neuralgia, tension-type headache, temporomandibular joint dysfunction, giant cell arteritis (also known as temporal arteritis) and medication overuse headache, as well as the trigeminal autonomic cephalalgias, including cluster headache, paroxysmal hemicrania, and hemicrania continua. Diagnostic criteria are discussed and evidence outlined that allows physicians to make better clinical diagnoses and point patients toward better treatment options.

Secondary headaches are classified by the cause of the underlying disease process that is causing the headache. There are hundreds of secondary headache diagnoses and this article is not an exhaustive discussion of secondary headache disorders. Maintaining a high level of virulence and having a structured approach to evaluating all patients with headache is the key to timely diagnosis of secondary headache disorders. Diagnostic testing is indicated based on the suspected disorder and management is determined by treatment of the underlying disease causing the headache.

This article clarifies the current state of knowledge of chronic oral, head, and facial pain (COHFP) conditions with the inclusion of temporomandibular joint disorders as just one component of the variety of conditions that can cause head and facial pain. Obtaining an accurate diagnosis in a timely manner is extremely important because COHFP symptoms can be caused by a variety of pathologic conditions that can be inflammatory, degenerative, neurologic, neoplastic, or systemic in origin. The essential role of the specialty of otolaryngology in the diagnosis and management of patients with these complex COHFP conditions is emphasized.

Vertiginous headache encompasses patients with dizziness or vertigo as well as headache, even though the symptoms may not occur in an obvious temporal relationship. The type of dizziness experienced by patients is different from the heavy-headedness experienced during rhinogenic headache. Patients may have a personal or family history of typical or atypical migraine. They should be evaluated for possible Meniere syndrome, migraine headaches, and/or eye movement disorders. Management is directed to treatment of the underlying abnormality. Long-term follow-up of these patients is necessary, because further otologic abnormalities may present later.

This article reviews the definition, etiology and evaluation, and medical and neurosurgical treatment of neuropathic facial pain. A neuropathic origin for facial pain should be considered when evaluating a patient for rhinologic surgery because of complaints of facial pain. Neuropathic facial pain is caused by vascular compression of the trigeminal nerve in the prepontine cistern and is characterized by an intermittent prickling or stabbing component or a constant burning, searing pain. Medical treatment consists of anticonvulsant medication. Neurosurgical treatment may require microvascular decompression of the trigeminal nerve.

OTOLARYNGOLOGIC CLINICS
OF NORTH AMERICA

NOW AVAILABLE FOR YOUR iPhone and iPad

Preface

Headache in Otolaryngology: Rhinogenic and Beyond

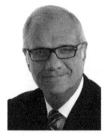 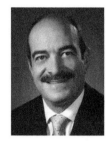

Howard Levine, MD   Michael Setzen, MD
Editors

Many patients present to their physicians with headache or mid facial pain and are certain that it is a "sinus headache." Specialists of all types, in particular, otolaryngologists, neurologists, allergists, internists, and emergency physicians, are confronted almost daily with patients saying, "Doc, I have a sinus headache and I need an antibiotic." This initiates a series of questions for the physician because several kinds of headaches occur with symptoms in this location. Also, the diagnosis is challenging because there are frequently associated symptoms of nasal congestion that accompany the headache and the common onset of headache with barometric change. Both of these symptom groups can be present in both sinus headaches and migraine.

"Headache in Otolaryngology: Rhinogenic and Beyond" describes headaches ascribed to other causes, in particular, migraine, as well as headaches that actually are a result of sinusitis. This issue addresses the need for the expertise of an otolaryngologist who can obtain a history of nasal and sinus disease, evaluate the interior of the nose, and correlate it to a computed tomographic scan, along with collaboration of neurologists/headache specialists. Because headaches are often a symptom of potentially dangerous conditions that may need emergency workup and referral to the appropriate physician, information in this issue identifies these emergency conditions for the clinician.

The approach to the subject of headache in this issue provides information of importance to not only otolaryngologists, but also emergency physicians, allergists, internists, pediatricians, pulmonologists, and family practitioners, who frequently see and manage headache and sinus patients. It provides direct clinical information on history, differential diagnosis, laboratory testing and imaging, and treatment options, along with suggestions for when to refer. It demonstrates the need for a multispecialty

Otolaryngol Clin N Am 47 (2014) xi–xii
http://dx.doi.org/10.1016/j.otc.2013.11.004
oto.theclinics.com

team approach in the evaluation of the headache patient, in particular, the patient reporting a "sinus headache" that can be anything *but* a sinus headache.

Howard Levine, MD
Acclarent, Inc
1525 O'Brien Drive
Menlo Park, CA 94025, USA

Michael Setzen, MD
NYU School of Medicine
Michael Setzen Otolaryngology, PC
600 Northern Boulevard, Suite 312
Great Neck, NY 11021, USA

E-mail addresses:
HLevine@ITS.JNJ.com (H. Levine)
michaelsetzen@gmail.com (M. Setzen)

Why the Confusion About Sinus Headache?

Howard Levine, MD[a],*, Michael Setzen, MD[b,c],
Chantal Holy, PhD[d]

KEYWORDS

- Sinus • Headache • Migraine • Treatment • MarketScan commercial database

KEY POINTS

- Symptoms of migraine headache and sinus headache can be similar.
- Both can occur with nasal congestion and facial pain, and can worsen during weather change.
- Sinus headache and the associated treatments can be found extensively in references on the Internet.

"Doctor, I have a sinus headache!" These words are heard frequently by physicians, especially otolaryngologists, headache specialists, neurologists, primary care physicians, pediatricians, and emergency room physicians. Although patients frequently believe they have a sinus problem, sinus headaches are not as common as individuals might think.

Some studies suggest that up to 90% of sinus headaches are actually migraines.[1,2] The confusion occurs partly because migraine headache involves activation of the trigeminal nerves that innervate both the sinus region and the meninges surrounding the brain. As a result, the site from which the pain originates is difficult to accurately determine. Additionally, nasal congestion can be a common feature of migraine headaches because of the autonomic nerve stimulation that can also cause tearing (lacrimation) and a runny nose (rhinorrhea). A study found that patients with sinus headaches responded to triptan migraine medications, but stated dissatisfaction with their

Disclosures: Employee of Acclarent, an Ethicon, Johnson & Johnson Company, Medical Affairs (H.L. Levine); Speaker's Bureau for Teva Pharmaceutical Industries Ltd and Meda Pharmaceuticals Inc (M. Setzen), this relationship has nothing to do with this publication; Employee of Acclarent, an Ethicon, Johnson & Johnson Company (C. Holy).
[a] Head and Neck Institute, The Cleveland Clinic, Cleveland, OH, USA; [b] Department of Otolaryngology, NYU Langone School of Medicine, New York, NY, USA; [c] Department of Rhinology, North Shore University Hospital at Manhasset, Manhasset, NY, USA; [d] Health Economics & Value Proposition, Acclarent, Inc, 1525-B O'Brien Drive, Menlo Park, CA 94025-1463, USA
* Corresponding author. Acclarent, Inc, 1525-B O'Brien Drive, Menlo Park, CA 94025-1463, USA
E-mail address: HLevine@ITS.JNJ.com

Otolaryngol Clin N Am 47 (2014) 169–174
http://dx.doi.org/10.1016/j.otc.2013.11.003
0030-6665/14/$ – see front matter © 2014 Elsevier Inc. All rights reserved.

treatment when they were treated with decongestants or antibiotics.[3] Treating these common symptoms without having the correct diagnosis can create overuse and misuse of resources, unnecessary surgeries, and unhappy patients. This issue addresses the differences and subtleties of sinus headaches.

To better understand the overall frequency of diagnosis, treatment pathways, and procedures and costs associated with sinus headaches, the Truven MarketScan (formerly Thomson Reuters) Commercial Claims and Encounters Database (Version 183), the largest United States–based claims database, was queried. MarketScan includes inpatient, outpatient, and prescription histories for all patients. For 2012 alone, MarketScan contains information on more than 50 million lives, with medical data available over multiple continuous years. This database is therefore extremely valuable, in that it can be used to track large patient cohorts longitudinally over time.

Because no specific International Classification of Diseases, Ninth Revision (ICD-9) diagnostic code exists for sinus headache, ICD-9 code 784.0 for headache (without further mention of cause or type) was used. This code is not specific to sinus headaches, but it provided the best match of all currently available diagnostic codes because it includes all headaches that are neither migraine/tension headache nor other forms of definable headache. Using this preliminary diagnosis code, a series of queries were built (**Fig. 1**) to understand how many of these headache diagnoses truly end up being caused by sinus disease. Specifically, all patients with a 784.0 diagnosis in the outpatient setting in January 2011 were identified. Of those, patients who also had a concurrent head computed tomography (CT) scan within ±30 days of the 784.0 diagnosis were further queried (**Table 1** provides a list of current procedural terminology used to identify head CTs), because these patients possibly underwent CT scan for sinus disease. The percentage of those patients with a 784.0 headache diagnosis and a sinus CT who were actually diagnosed with acute sinusitis, chronic sinusitis, or polyposis within 3 months of their CT was then analyzed. To do so, this subset of patients with an ICD-9 diagnosis code of 461.X (acute sinusitis), 473.X (chronic sinusitis), or 471.X (polyposis) were queried (the "X" means that all ICD-9 with the first 3 digits as shown here and any possible 4th digit were included).

A total cohort of 83,868 cases was identified (100%). Of those, 13,752 underwent a sinus CT. Within these 13,752 patients, only 3214 had a subsequent diagnosis of either sinusitis or polyposis (23.4% of patients with CT or 3.8% of the entire headache cohort).

This analysis, although not perfect because the headache diagnosis was not specific to sinus headache, does confirm anecdotal reports of overuse of "sinus headache." In addition, the findings suggest that, when migraine and all other causes of headaches are dismissed, only a small fraction of patients actually experience sinus headache ($\approx$3.8%). This percentage correlates with other reports. A total of 100 patients who self-reported sinus headache were found after evaluation to have a variety of headaches (migraine, 63%; probable migraine, 23%; unclassifiable, 9%; hemicranias continua, 1%; cluster, 1%; and sinus headache, 3%).[4]

The MarketScan Outpatient View analysis provided some understanding of the overall costs associated with this broad headache diagnosis (ICD-9 784.0), and although most cases may not be sinus headaches per se, these diagnoses represent a significant burden for patients, providers, and payers. Specifically, in 2012, there were 13.5 million patient visits during which a patient was diagnosed with a 784.0 code. Nearly 20% of these were assigned in the emergency room and 66% were assigned in the physician's office. Of all diagnoses, 70% were given to female patients. The total expenses paid for these episodes were estimated at

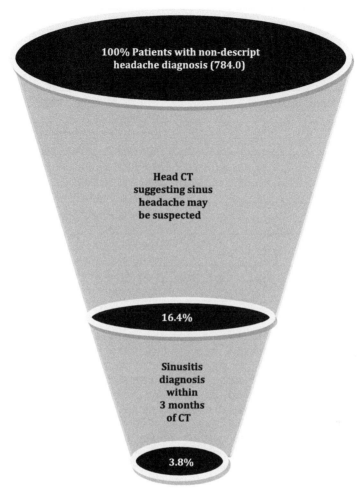

100% Patients with non-descript headache diagnosis (784.0)

Head CT suggesting sinus headache may be suspected

16.4%

Sinusitis diagnosis within 3 months of CT

3.8%

Fig. 1. Of all patients presenting with a nonmigraine, nonexplainable headache (ICD-9 784.0), 16.4% obtain a head CT, and of these patients, fewer than 1 in 4 will be diagnosed with sinusitis or polyposis within 3 months of their CT.

$892 million: $567 million by commercial payers and $117 by Medicare, and the remainder being paid through Medicaid and private pay. Of all 13.5 million visits, 624,980 were to otolaryngologists. Although non–sinus-specific, of the 13.5 million episodes, one can estimate based on the numbers mentioned that 16.4% of the patients experiencing these episodes may be given a sinus CT at a per-unit payment of $377 (payment analysis of CTs performed specifically on patients experiencing sinus disease and before sinus surgery, using MarketScan), and of these, fewer than 1 in 4 will end up having sinusitis or polyposis. This short analysis, with all its imperfections and assumptions, highlights the significant challenge and cost associated with accurately diagnosing sinus headaches.

CASE EXAMPLE

A 34-year-old primary school teacher visits her otolaryngologist with concerns about sinusitis and headaches. Sinusitis occurs several times a year. Each episode lasts

Table 1	
Current procedural terminology used to identify head CTs, possibly associated with sinusitis	
70496	CT angiography, head
70540	MRI orbit/face/neck without dye
70542	MRI orbit/face/neck with dye
70543	MRI orbit/face/neck with and without dye
70544	MR angiography head without dye
70545	MR angiography head with dye
70546	MR angiography head with and without dye
70450	CT head/brain without dye
70460	CT head/brain with dye
70470	CT head/brain with and without dye
70480	CT orbit/ear/fossa without dye
70481	CT orbit/ear/fossa with dye
70482	CT orbit/ear/fossa with and without dye
70486	CT maxillofacial without dye
70487	CT maxillofacial with dye
70488	CT maxillofacial with and without dye

from a day or so to a week or more. The episodes are manifest by nasal obstruction, clear or discolored nasal drainage, nasal congestion, and mid face or forehead pain. The facial pain and pressure can range from mild to severe, and be accompanied by throbbing and nausea. The episodes often begin with a cold, sore throat, and cough and progress to thick discolored nasal drainage. Each episode may begin with a weather change and/or air travel. The patient's dentist noted something on the floor of one maxillary sinus on routine dental films. Over-the-counter sinus medications have helped her symptoms. When they do not provide relief, her primary care physician prescribes a 5-day antibiotic, which often helps. When asked, the patient describes 2 types of headaches. One type occurs several times a year, and another occurs almost every month. The head pain that occurs several times a year is associated with the cough and sore throat. She sometimes experiences some sick feeling in the stomach with the monthly headaches. The facial pain and headache can be a pressure or throbbing type of pain, and occasionally can be severe. Her family history includes a mother who has a history of headaches and a father who has undergone sinus surgery for sinusitis.

DISCUSSION

This patient's history is common to the otolaryngologist. The patient assumes all her symptoms and episodes are from sinusitis. She believes this because of the frequency, location of the pain, associated nasal symptoms, radiographic evidence by the dentist of something in the sinus, improvement with sinus medications, and a family history of headache and sinusitis. This patient may have recurrent acute sinusitis possibly caused by occupational exposure to various infections acquired in the classroom. The patient expects to be "cured" of the all of the symptoms, because she believes it is from sinusitis, and because both the Internet and the media claim that this headache is a sinus headache caused by sinusitis and can be readily treated with sinus medication. However, a careful understanding of the signs and symptoms would lead to a diagnosis of recurrent acute sinusitis or migraine, or a combination of both. Although those diagnoses might seem obvious to the reader and practitioner, establishing the diagnosis might be more complicated in other patients. For this patient and others like her, it is important to treat the sinusitis and also to educate the patient about the different types of headaches and similarity of symptoms. This information will allow the patient to know when to accurately treat each of the separate problems. This similarity among headaches, however, frequently poses a challenge, because many patients are convinced their symptoms are sinus in origin. Cases like this pose a challenge and confusion to all involved, including the patient and the health professional.

Many other factors contribute to the confusion about sinus headache. This confusion is caused by not only the similarity of signs and symptoms but also the media and pharmaceutical companies recommending numerous medications for sinus headache as being effective. An Internet search produces more than 2 million responses for the key phrase "sinus headache treatment." WebMD lists more than 150 over-the-counter medications that can be used to treat sinus headache. Many of these medications contain an analgesic, and patients believe that because their headache is improved by the sinus medication, sinusitis is the cause. However, the positive response is more from the analgesic than from any of the other active ingredients to treat sinusitis.

In addition, an Internet search for "natural remedies for sinus headache" produced more than 261,000 results. Although Internet search results may not be exact, they do show the scope and volume of information available on the Internet for treating "sinus headache."

Even the 2013 International Classification of Headache[5] is uncertain of its definitions of sinus headache. It states that the term "sinus headache" is outmoded because it refers to both primary and secondary headache.

It is easy for patients and physicians to be confused about the symptoms and signs related to facial pain, pressure, and headache associated with sinus disease. The typical symptoms of headache from acute sinusitis include worsening with weather change, nasal obstruction, and congestion and discolored or clear nasal drainage. Despite this definition, all of these symptoms can be caused by acute sinusitis or migraine headache. Migraine headaches have a vascular component and can cause the congestion and nasal obstruction. Even physical examination of the nasal cavity can produce confusion. Congestion seen within the nose can be from primary nasal or sinus disorder or from the vascular component of a migraine headache. Furthermore, even a CT scan showing thickening of the mucous membrane of the sinus cannot confirm headache caused by acute sinusitis or migraine. Nasal congestion and/or obstruction may be secondary to the vascular component of the migraine headache or acute sinusitis.

SUMMARY

Sinus headache is usually caused by migraine, and rarely by rhinogenic causes. The correct diagnosis can be rewarding to both the practitioner and a happy well-served patient. Understanding the cause of the headache will lead to the correct medical or surgical treatment, and allow management of the sinuses with traditional techniques or newer minimally invasive approaches.[6] Through understanding and listening to the patient's history, the correct diagnosis can be usually made, enabling optimal treatment. This issue of the *Otolaryngologic Clinics of North America* will contribute to a better understanding of the dilemma.

REFERENCES

1. Schreiber C, Hutchinson S, Webster C, et al. Prevalence of migraine in patients with a history of self-reported or physician-diagnosed "sinus" headache. Arch Intern Med 2004;164(16):1769–72. http://dx.doi.org/10.1001/archinte.164.16.1769.
2. Mehle ME, Schreiber CP. Sinus headache, migraine, and the otolaryngologist. Otolaryngol Head Neck Surg 2005;133(4):489–96. http://dx.doi.org/10.1016/j.otohns.2005.05.659.
3. Ishkanian G, Blumenthal H, Webster CJ, et al. Efficacy of sumatriptan tablets in migraineurs self-described or physician-diagnosed as having sinus headache: a randomized, double-blind, placebo-controlled study. Clin Ther 2007;29(1):99–109.
4. Erross EJ. Poster presented at the International Headache Congress. Rome, Italy, September 13–16, 2003.
5. Headache Classification Subcommittee of the International Headache Society. The international classification of headache disorders: 2nd edition. Cephalalgia 2004;24(Suppl 1):9–160.
6. Marzetti A, Tedaldi M, Passali FM. The role of balloon sinuplasty in the treatment of sinus headache. Otolaryngol Pol, in press.

Diagnosing and Understanding Adult Headache

Alexander Feoktistov, MD, PhD, Merle Diamond, MD*

KEYWORDS

- Migraine • Tension-type headache • Cluster headache

KEY POINTS

- Primary headache disorders are the most common forms of headaches.
- Taking a good history and performing thorough physical and neurologic examination are mandatory in evaluation of patients with headache.
- Unusual age of onset, sudden change in the headache pattern, headache deterioration, and lack of response to therapy, as well as presence of systemic symptoms such as fever and weight loss should warrant further diagnostic work-up.

Headaches are among the most frequent reasons for patients to seek medical attention and one of the largest contributors to disability. It is one of the most common disorders of nervous system.[1] Primary headaches are the most common forms of headache disorders.

Primary headaches represent idiopathic pain conditions without underlying disorders, whereas secondary headaches disorders occur because of another pathologic process.

There are more than 17 different types of primary headache disorders with the most common being tension-type headache, migraines, and cluster headaches. Examples of secondary headache disorders are injury-related or trauma-related headaches, headaches secondary to infections, vascular disorders, and tumors (**Table 1**).

With some variations, primary headaches occur in all age groups, affecting people of different races and geographic locations as well as different income levels, thus representing a global problem. It has been reported that 47% of the general adult population worldwide experienced at least a single headache episode in the past year,[1] whereas 1.7% to 4% of the adult population worldwide has been experienced chronic headaches (at least 15 headache days per month). According to the 2010 Global Burden of Disease Study, worldwide prevalence of tension-type headache was

Disclosures: None.
Diamond Headache Clinic, 1460 North Halsted Street, Suite 501, Chicago, IL 60642, USA
* Corresponding author.
E-mail address: mdiamond@diamondheadache.com

Table 1	
Primary and secondary headache disorders	
Primary Headache	**Secondary Headache**
Tension-type headache	Headache attributed to trauma or injury to the head or neck
Migraine	Headache attributed to cranial or cervical vascular disorder
Trigeminal autonomic cephalalgias	Headache attributed to a substance or its withdrawal
Primary exercise headaches	Headache attributed to infection
Primary stabbing headaches	Headache attributed to disorder or homeostasis
New daily persistent headache	Headache attributed to psychiatric disorder
Hypnic headache	Painful cranial neuropathies and other facial pains

From International Headache Society. International Classification of Headache Disorders, 3rd edition-beta. Cephalalgia 2013;33(9):627–808; with permission.

estimated to be 20% and migraine more than 14%, placing them in second and third places respectively among the most common disorders in the world.[2] It has been estimated that migraine contributed to 2.9% of all years of life lost to disability, ranking it as number 7 among the most disabling disorders.[2]

TENSION-TYPE HEADACHE

Tension-type headache is the most common primary headache disorder worldwide. Because tension-type headache is less severe and less disabling, it is seen less frequently in clinical practice. It has been estimated that 1-year prevalence of tension-type headache is 63% in men and 83% in women.[3] Pathophysiology of tension-type headache is still poorly understood. A previously considered psychogenic cause does not reflect or explain all aspects of tension-type headache. It is currently thought that tension-type headaches have a strong neurobiological basis.[4] At present, it is considered that peripheral pain mechanisms are involved in infrequent tension-type headache pathogenesis and central pain mechanisms in the chronic form. Presence of pericranial myofascial tenderness suggests the participation of central pain mechanisms, including possible sensitization at the level of dorsal horn and trigeminal nucleus caudalis.[5] Because many patients with tension-type headache show symptoms of migraines (such as occasional presence of headache with a throbbing quality, and response to triptans), some specialist think that tension-type headache represents the opposite of the migraine end of the headache spectrum.

Tension-type headaches are subcategorized into 4 main categories: infrequent (less than 1 day per month), frequent (1–14 headache days per month for more than 3 month), chronic (more than 15 headache days per month for more than 3 months), and probable tension-type headache. The first 3 subcategories are also divided into tension-type headache associated with pericranial tenderness and those not associated with pericranial tenderness, which should be confirmed during physical examination (**Box 1**).

Tension-type headache usually presents as mild to moderate, dull, pressurelike pain located in the forehead, in the occipital area. The pain is usually located bilaterally. Patients frequently describe tension-type headache as a rubber band–like sensation around the head. In more severe cases of tension-type headache, the pain has a throbbing or pulsating quality and may even be associated with either photophobia

---

Box 1
Classification of tension-type headache

2. Tension-type headache

   2.1. Infrequent episodic tension-type headache

      2.1.1. Infrequent episodic tension-type headache associated with pericranial tenderness

      2.1.2. Infrequent episodic tension-type headache not associated with pericranial tenderness

   2.2. Frequent episodic tension-type headache

      2.2.1. Frequent episodic tension-type headache associated with pericranial tenderness

      2.2.2. Frequent episodic tension-type headache not associated with pericranial tenderness

   2.3. Chronic tension-type headache

      2.3.1. Chronic tension-type headache associated with pericranial tenderness

      2.3.2. Chronic tension-type headache not associated with pericranial tenderness

   2.4. Probable tension-type headache

      2.4.1. Probable infrequent episodic tension-type headache

      2.4.2. Probable frequent episodic tension-type headache

      2.4.3. Probable chronic tension-type headache

From International Headache Society. International Classification of Headache Disorders, 3rd edition-beta. Cephalalgia 2013;33(9):627–808; with permission.

---

or phonophobia, which may represent a challenge in differentiating tension-type headache from a mild form of migraine without aura. Tension-type headache may last from 30 minutes to 7 days and usually is not aggravated by routine physical activity (**Box 2**). Some patients obtain relief while participating in low-grade physical activity.

Case Presentation

A 42-year-old female advertising executive complains of intermittent headache. The pain is located bifrontally and she describes it as a pressure-like sensation. The headache is not associated with nausea or sensitivity to light or noise. She states that she is usually able to maintain her routine activities, although she feels fatigued most of the time. These headaches date back 5 years and have occurred weekly for the past 8 months. They frequently seem to be provoked by work-related stress. Physical examination revealed that the pericranial muscles were tender to palpation. The rest of the physical and neurologic examination, as well as results of blood work, were unremarkable.

The diagnosis was of frequent episodic tension-type headache associated with pericranial tenderness.

Clinical presentation of this case is typical for tension-type headache. Presence of systemic symptoms such as generalized fatigue should warrant further work-up. Differential diagnosis in this case should include hypothyroidism, anemia, fibromyalgia, and sinusitis. Absence of fever, nasal congestion especially with purulent discharge, and normal laboratory findings make diagnosis of sinusitis less likely. In addition, performing route blood work (including erythrocyte sedimentation rate, complete blood

> **Box 2**
> **Diagnostic criteria of infrequent tension-type headache**
>
> A. At least 10 episodes of headache occurring on fewer than 1 day per month on average (<12 days per year) and fulfilling criteria B to D
>
> B. Lasting from 30 minutes to 7 days
>
> C. At least 2 of the following 4 characteristics:
>   - Bilateral location
>   - Pressing or tightening (none pulsating) quality
>   - Mild or moderate intensity
>   - Not aggravated by routine physical activities such as walking or climbing stairs
>
> D. Both of the following:
>   - No nausea or vomiting
>   - No more than 1 of phonophobia or photophobia
>
> E. Not better accounted for by another International Classification of Headache Disorders, 3rd edition (ICDH-3) diagnosis
>
> *From* International Headache Society. International Classification of Headache Disorders, 3rd edition-beta. Cephalalgia 2013;33(9):627–808; with permission.

count, complete metabolic profile, and thyroid-stimulating hormone) should be helpful in making the correct diagnosis. Absence of chronic diffuse generalized myofascial pain makes diagnosis of fibromyalgia unlikely.

MIGRAINE

Migraine is the second most common primary headache disorder (tension-type headache being the first) and it is the most common diagnosis among people with headache seeking medical attention. It affects 18% of all women and 6% of all men in the United States.[6]

Although migraine affects different age groups it most commonly occurs between the ages of 35 and 45 years, which seem to be the most productive years. Thus the economic impact should not be overlooked.[7] Direct cost of migraine treatment encounters for US$1 billion per year in the United States alone. Total economic impact of the loss of productivity caused by migraines is estimated at US$13 billion per year.[8]

Pathophysiologic mechanisms of migraine are complex and consist of the involvement of cerebral blood vessels, venous sinuses, trigeminal nerve, upper cervical dorsal roots, and the genetically predisposed hyperexcitability of these systems, and they involve activation of the pain-producing structures (trigeminocervical complex), release of calcitonin gene–related peptide, substance P, and nitric oxide, which lead to vasodilatation, plasma protein extravasation, and sterile neurogenic inflammation, which in turn further promote central sensitization and trigeminocervical system activation.[9]

Migraine headaches are divided in to 2 major groups: migraine with and without aura (see **Box 1**).[10] They can be further subdivided into episodic and chronic forms (>15 headache days per month for at least 3 months). There are also complications of migraine such as status migrainosus, and persistent aura without infarction (**Box 3**).

Migraine classically presents as unilateral pain located in the temple region. In practice, migraine may present as bitemporal or even global headache involving the entire

---

Box 3
Migraine classification

1. Migraine
   1.1. Migraine without aura
   1.2. Migraine with aura
       1.2.1. Migraine with typical aura
           1.2.1.1. Typical aura with headache
           1.2.1.2. Typical aura without headache
       1.2.2. Migraine with brainstem aura
       1.2.3. Hemiplegic migraine
           1.2.3.1. Familial hemiplegic migraine
               1.2.3.1.1. Familial hemiplegic migraine type 1
               1.2.3.1.2. Familial hemiplegic migraine type 2
               1.2.3.1.3. Familial hemiplegic migraine type 3
               1.2.3.1.4. Familial hemiplegic migraine, other loci
           1.2.3.2. Sporadic hemiplegic migraine
       1.2.4. Retinal migraine
   1.3. Chronic migraine
   1.4. Complications of migraine
       1.4.1. Status migrainosus
       1.4.2. Persistent aura without infarction
       1.4.3. Migrainosus infarction
       1.4.4. Migraine aura-triggered seizure
   1.5. Probable migraine
       1.5.1. Probable migraine without aura
       1.5.2. Probable migraine with aura
   1.6. Episodic syndromes that may be associated with migraine
       1.6.1. Recurrent gastrointestinal disturbance
           1.6.1.1. Cyclic vomiting syndrome
           1.6.1.2. Abdominal migraine
       1.6.2. Benign paroxysmal vertigo
       1.6.3. Benign paroxysmal torticollis

From International Headache Society. International Classification of Headache Disorders, 3rd edition-beta. Cephalalgia 2013;33(9):627–808; with permission.

---

head. Patients often start experiencing pain unilaterally and, as pain progresses, it may either migrate to the opposite side or transform into a bilateral global headache. The pain is most often rated by patients as moderate to severe and disabling, and associated with photophobia and phonophobia as well as nausea and vomiting. Most of the patients need to stop or at least significantly reduce their activity during a severe migraine attack and confine themselves to a dark, quiet room. Migraine usually lasts between 4 and 72 hours, with the most common duration being 24 hours if untreated. Migraine headache is characteristically associated with nausea and/or vomiting. Presence of at least one of these associated symptoms is important to a diagnosis (**Box 4**). Some patients also experience elements of cutaneous allodynia before or during a migraine attack.[10] As stated previously, migraine headache usually begins in childhood or the teenage years and may persist throughout most of the patient's life.

About 20% of all patients with migraine headaches experience migraine aura. Aura represents brief (usually lasting between 5 and 60 minutes) and either simple neurologic phenomena, such as visual changes (negative or positive scotoma, visual field distortion, photopsias and so forth), sensory abnormality (unilateral paresthesia or numbness), and aphasia. In some rare instances, migraine aura may present as more complex and complicated neurologic phenomena such as hemiplegia (as in hemiplegic migraines) or vertigo, double vision, and/or bilateral paresthesia, as seen in migraines with brain stem aura, which should warrant more careful and thorough diagnostic approach and frequently should involve imaging. An important characteristic of migraine aura is that it is temporary and reversible even in the absence of treatment (see **Box 4**).

Physical examination and laboratory findings are usually unremarkable. Imaging (either magnetic resonance imaging [MRI] of the brain with and without contrast or computed tomography scan of the head) is not always warranted but is frequently performed to rule out intracranial disorders (tumors, infections, trauma, and so forth), especially in the right clinical setting. Performance of magnetic resonance angiography [MRA] of the head and neck may be necessary when a vascular disorder (aneurism, arterial dissection, and so forth) is suspected. Migraine is a primary headache disorder, so imaging and other diagnostic tests are expected to be negative and diagnostic tests should be used not to diagnose migraine headache but to rule out other disorders.

The usual warning signs that trigger a physician's interest in further investigations are presence of fever, weight loss, strictly unilateral location of headache without

---

Box 4
Migraine diagnostic criteria

A. At least 5 attacks fulfilling criteria A to D

B. Headache attack lasting 4 to 72 hours (untreated or unsuccessfully treated)

C. Headache has at least 2 of the following 4 characteristics:

    a. Unilateral location

    b. Pulsating quality

    c. Moderate or severe pain intensity

    d. Aggravation by or causing avoidance of routine physical activity

D. During headache at least 1 of the following:

    • Nausea or/and vomiting

    • Phonophobia and photophobia

E. Not better accounted for by another ICDH-3 diagnosis

From International Headache Society. International Classification of Headache Disorders, 3rd edition-beta. Cephalalgia 2013;33(9):627–808; with permission.

history of headache involving the other side or another part of the head, unusual (especially late) age of onset of migraines, prolonged or unusual neurologic symptoms (aura), lack of response to treatment, or changing pain pattern.

Case Presentation

A 24-year-old woman complains of recurrent severe throbbing headache usually located on one side of the head. She states that the duration of the headache varies but it usually lasts 24 hours. The headache is almost always associated with nausea, occasionally vomiting, and sensitivity to light and noise to the extent that she prefers to stay in a dark and quiet room. She also states that during severe headache she is not able to function or maintain her routine daily activity and that any physical activity makes her headache worse. She also notices increased fatigue and yawning, irritability, and food craving within a day before the headache. She states that occasionally she sees flashing lights or experiences facial numbness that usually last for a few minutes and then disappear. She states that she started experiencing these headaches in her teenage years. The patient's mother has also been having infrequent migraines. Physical and neurologic examinations are normal.

The diagnosis was of migraine with aura.

This case involves a young woman with history of throbbing headaches going back to her teenage years: the history that is frequently seen in patients with migraine. The associated symptoms and prodrome described in this case are also typical for migraine headaches. She has a positive history of migraine headache in her mother. She describes a phenomenon of visual and sensory aura that precedes migraine and the visual and sensory changes that she is describing are completely reversible. In this case, there is no need for imaging because this patient has classic migraine presentations and her neurologic examination is normal, although this could be reconsidered if she develops new or unusual symptoms.

Next case is another patient with frequent recurrent severe headaches that are in contrast with the previous case.

Case Presentation

A 44-year-old woman without significant past medical history presented with a 2-year history of severe headaches. She described her headaches as being initially episodic but progressively worsening. She reported that the headache intensity was severe and that the pain location varied and could be either unilateral or bilateral. She described the pain as throbbing in nature and associated with nausea, vomiting, photophobia, and phonophobia. She was diagnosed with migraine without aura 6 months ago by her primary care physician and she was treated with nonsteroidal antiinflammatory drugs with minimal relief and later with triptans, β-blockers, topiramate, and venlafaxine. In the past 2 months she noticed that coughing and sneezing aggravated the headache. She eventually developed an episode of severe throbbing headache with intractable vomiting and with the diagnosis of status migrainosus she was admitted for rehydration and parenteral pain management. Physical and neurologic examinations were unremarkable. Laboratory data were positive for signs of dehydration. MRI brain was done, which revealed approximately six 5-cm frontal lobe meningiomas (Fig. 1).

As seen from this case, clinical presentation of headache resembles migraine especially if considered outside the case context. The worrisome signs in this case are late age of onset; the patient started experiencing her headaches at the age of 42 years, which is an unusual age of initial migraine presentation. Another suspicious clinical pattern is progressively worsening headaches and lack of response to acute and

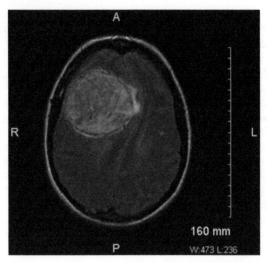

Fig. 1. Meningioma.

preventative treatment modalities. Thus, this presentation shows that, even in the absence of distinct neurologic signs (mental status change, paralysis, aphasia, and so forth), it is important to analyze and take into diagnostic consideration the entire presentation, including past medical history and history of present illness.

Overall, headaches attributed to tumors are uncommon (less than 5% of all cases with headaches), but about 20% of patients with intracranial mass lesions present with headache as their initial symptoms, and 60% of patients develop headache during the course of the illness. Eighty-two percent of patients notice change in the preexisting headache pattern with tumor occurrence.

CLUSTER HEADACHE

Cluster headache is the most severe primary headache disorder. One of the nicknames of cluster headaches used to be suicide headache, reflecting the severity and intractability of this disorder. Cluster headaches are less common than migraine or tension-type headache, with an estimated overall prevalence of 0.2%. They occur more frequently in men, with male/female right ratio being between 3:1 and 6:1. Cluster headaches are classified as one of the subtypes of trigeminal autonomic cephalalgias (TACs), and are further subdivided into episodic and chronic forms (**Box 5**).

Box 5
Classification of cluster headache

3. TACs

    3.1. Cluster headache

        3.1.1. Episodic cluster headache

        3.1.2. Chronic cluster headache

From International Headache Society. International Classification of Headache Disorders, 3rd edition-beta. Cephalalgia 2013;33(9):627–808; with permission.

The pathogenesis of cluster headache is complex. Activation of the ipsilateral hypothalamus was noted on positron emission tomography imaging during acute cluster attacks. Furthermore, deep brain stimulation applied to these regions produced rapid symptom cessation. Hypothalamic involvement has been hypothesized for many years because of the rhythmicity of cluster attacks and because the suprachiasmatic nucleus of the hypothalamus plays an important role in the regulation of human circadian rhythms. Parasympathetic hyperactivity has also been implicated in cluster headache pathogenesis, which explains the presence of lacrimation, rhinorrhea, conjunctival injection, and nasal congestion. The reasons for parasympathetic hyperactivity are still poorly understood.[11]

Cluster headaches are typically described as sharp, boring, burning, or stabbing pain located retro-orbitally or in the temporal region. They are regarded as a strictly unilateral headache disorder with little variability in location of the pain from attack to attack.[7] Cases have been described in which cluster headaches switch sides between different cluster cycles but more commonly the pain remains locked to the same location/side. Typical cluster attacks last from 15 to 180 minutes. Patients tend to experience multiple attacks in a 24-hour period with headaches frequently occurring in the middle of the night. The pain is characteristically associated with ptosis, nasal congestion or rhinorrhea, ipsilateral lacrimation, and/or conjunctival injection (**Box 6**). Cluster headache attacks are usually grouped in cluster cycles with each cycle lasting from several weeks to several months. Cluster cycles tend to occur more frequently during the spring and fall. Patients may have fewer symptoms for months to several years between different cluster cycles (as with episodic cluster headache) or may experience daily clusters attacks for many years (as with patients with chronic cluster headache).

Box 6
Diagnostic criteria of cluster headache

A. At least 5 attacks fulfilling criteria B to D

B. Severe or very severe unilateral orbital, supraorbital and/or temporal pain lasting 15 to 180 minutes

C. Either or both of the following:

1. At least 1 of the following symptoms or signs, ipsilateral to the headache:
   - Conjunctival injection and/or lacrimation
   - Nasal congestion and/or rhinorrhea
   - Eyelid edema
   - Forehead and facial sweating
   - Forehead and facial flushing
   - Sensation of fullness in the ear
   - Miosis and/or ptosis
2. A sense of restlessness or agitation

D. Attacks have a frequency between 1 every other day and 8 per day for more than half of the time when the disorder is active

E. Not better accounted for by another ICDH-3 diagnosis

From International Headache Society. International Classification of Headache Disorders, 3rd edition-beta. Cephalalgia 2013;33(9):627–808; with permission.

Case Presentation

A 56-year-old man with insignificant past medical history and social history positive for smoking 1 pack per day for the past 30 years or more complains of severe, sharp, stabbing, burning pain behind his left eye. He rates the severity of the pain as 10 out of 10 on a visual analog scale. Duration of each attack is approximately 45 to 60 minutes if untreated and it is associated with left eye conjunctival injection, lacrimation, and left-sided nasal congestion. The patient denies any fever or chills and states that the headache frequently wakes him up in the middle of the night. He experiences up to 8 painful episodes per day. He started having these headaches 12 years ago. The headache seems to be occurring in cycles, with each cycle lasting 6 weeks. He may experience 2 cycles each year, typically in May and October. His physical examination and laboratory data were unremarkable. The MRI of the brain that was performed 4 years ago was negative.

The diagnosis was of episodic cluster headache.

Diagnosis of cluster headache is rarely challenging, but other clinical possibilities should be considered in differential diagnosis. Disorders such as temporal arteritis should be excluded considering that both of these conditions frequently occur in elderly individuals. Both conditions present with strictly unilateral pain location. Physical examination revealing tenderness of the temporal artery in temporal arteritis as well as laboratory data (highly increased erythrocyte sedimentation rate) should be helpful. Other differential diagnostic entities that should be considered are carotid or vertebral artery dissection, acute sinusitis, glaucoma, and intracranial aneurism. Careful history taking and thorough physical examination help in making the correct diagnosis. In more complicated cases, neuroimaging (MRI, MRA, or computed tomography angiography of the brain and neck) to rule out arterial dissection and aneurism may be necessary.

SUMMARY

Primary headache disorders represent the most common headache forms. Most of the primary headache disorders, although they may have typical characteristics, represent diagnoses of exclusion. Thorough history, physical examination, and more sophisticated diagnostic methods (including neuroimaging) should be used in suspicious cases.

REFERENCES

1. Available at: http://www.who.int/mediacentre/factsheets/fs277/en/.
2. Vos T, Flaxman AD, Naghavi M, et al. Years lived with disability (YLD) for 1160 sequelae of 289 diseases and injuries 1990–2010: a systematic analysis for the Global Burden of Disease Study 2010. Lancet 2012;14:2163–96.
3. Rasmussen BK. Epidemiology of headache. Cephalalgia 1995;15:45–68.
4. Ashina M. Neurobiology of chronic tension-type headache. Cephalalgia 2004;24:161–72.
5. Bendtsen L. Central sensitization in tension-type headache – possible pathophysiological mechanisms. Cephalalgia 2000;20:486–508.
6. Lipton RB, Stewart WF, Reed M, et al. Migraine's impact today. Burden of illness, patterns of care. Postgrad Med 2001;109:38–45.
7. Stewart WF, Lipton RB, Celentano DD, et al. Prevalence of migraine in the United States. Relation to age, income, race and other sociodemographic factors. JAMA 1992;267:64–9.

8. Hu XH, Markson LE, Lipton RB, et al. Burden of migraine in the United States: disability and economic costs. Arch Intern Med 1999;159:813–8.
9. Goadsby P, Edvinsson L, Ekman R. Release of vasoactive peptides in the extracerebral circulation of man and the cat during activation of the trigeminovascular system. Ann Neurol 1988;28:183–7.
10. Headache Classification Committee of the International Headache Society (IHS). International classification of headache disorders, 3rd edition-beta. Cephalalgia 2013;33(9):627–808.
11. Goadsby PJ. Pathophysiology of cluster headache: a trigeminal autonomic cephalgia. Lancet Neurol 2001;1:251–7.

Imaging for Headache
What the Otolaryngologist Looks for

Raza Pasha, MD[a,]*, Rafay Qamer Soleja[b], Mohammad Nadir Ijaz[c]

KEYWORDS

- Rhinogenic headache • Imaging • Contact-point headache
- Computed tomography • Otolaryngology • Sinusitis

KEY POINTS

- Rhinogenic causes of facial pain and headache in the absence of chronic or acute changes within the paranasal sinuses are challenging to identify strictly through imaging studies.
- Computed tomographic (CT) imaging findings of various degrees of paranasal sinus mucosal thickening may suggest a rhinogenic source for headaches and facial pain.
- CT findings suggesting a rhinogenic source of a headache often include subtle mucosal contacts, such as septal spurs or large lateral nasal structures.
- Anatomic variants that obstruct the outflow tracts of the paranasal sinuses, including reduction of the infundibular space, may also suggest a potential rhinologic source of facial pain.
- Identifying anatomic variants may help determine possible therapeutic procedures to treat a rhinogenic headache.

INTRODUCTION

The diagnostic criteria and standard of care for the management of acute, subacute, and chronic rhinosinusitis have been largely defined.[1-3] Embedded in these definitions are diagnostic imaging criteria that indicate mucosal disease within the paranasal sinuses.[1-3] These mucosal findings are elementary to identify, even for a non–head and neck trained physician or radiologist. Nonetheless, other rhinogenic sources of headache and facial pain have been debated in the literature and within rhino-logic circles. These rhinogenic sources include mucosal contact-point headaches,

The authors have no disclosures or conflicts of interest.
[a] Pasha Snoring and Sinus Center, 12121 Richmond Avenue, Suite 304, Houston, TX 77082, USA;
[b] University of Texas Medical Branch, 310 Watercrest Harbor Lane, League City, TX 77573, USA;
[c] 9717 Cypresswood Drive Apartment 2002, Houston, TX 77070, USA
* Corresponding author.
E-mail address: rpasha@PashaMD.com

Abbreviations	
ARS	Acute rhinosinusitis
CT	Computed tomography
FP	Facial pain
HA	Headache
HIV	Human immunodeficiency virus
OMC	Osteomeatal complex
RARS	Recurrent acute rhinosinusitis
TMJ	Temporomandibular joint
URI	Upper respiratory infection

barosinusitis, recurrent barotrauma, and recurrent acute rhinosinusitis (RARS). The diagnoses for these other potential sources may be challenging for clinicians because the patient may present with a normal examination or computed tomography (CT) scan between active episodes.[4,5]

In the absence of mucosal involvement, differentiating a rhinogenic from a nonrhinogenic source, such as a tension headache, migraine headache, temporomandibular joint disease, or cluster headaches through history and physical examination may be difficult. Imaging studies may only suggest a contact or obstruction point but are not hallmark to a particular rhinogenic headache diagnosis.[4–7] RARS poses a diagnostic dilemma in providing objective, radiographic findings in between acute episodes that can differentiate it from an upper respiratory infection.[6]

More complicated, and not covered in this review, are discussions regarding the potential of rhinogenic triggers that at least theoretically may elicit a classic cascade of physical events that lead to a migraine-variant–type headache.

This article focuses on CT findings associated with rhinogenic causes of headache and facial pain. These more advanced observations of CT scan variants will provide otolaryngologists with an additional tool besides clinical examination to diagnose and potentially treat rhinogenic headaches.

DEFINITIONS

Traditionally, rhinogenic headaches are defined as a headache or facial pain caused by a rhinologic source, yet this definition excludes classic acute and chronic sinusitis findings such as inflammatory sinonasal disease, nasal discharge, nasal polyps, nasal mass, hyperplastic mucosa, and tumors or foreign bodies.[8] This definition also excludes neurologic, neuromuscular, and vascular-type of headaches, including intracerebral causes, tension headaches, migraine headaches, temporomandibular joint disease, and cluster headaches. Mucosal contact-point headaches are a subset of rhinogenic headaches that are triggered by mucosal contact, most commonly from the lateral nasal wall to the septum.

According to the Rhinosinusitis Task Force, RARS is defined as 4 or more episodes of rhinosinusitis per year, but these episodes do not meet the duration criteria of more than 12 weeks to be considered chronic rhinosinusitis, and complete resolution of symptoms occurs between episodes.[1–3] Barosinusitis, whether active or recurrent, results in facial pain classically caused by descent from altitude or descent when diving.[9,10] When ventilation of the sinus outflow tract is inadequate or completely obstructed, a marked increase in pressure within the sinuses results in pain, and possibly mucosal inflammatory changes.

SYMPTOM CRITERIA

The Rhinosinusitis Task Force has differentiated RARS from acute rhinosinusitis as being characterized by 4 or more episodes of acute rhinosinusitis per year (**Table 1**).[7] Other potential rhinogenic triggers involving the paranasal sinus that are associated with absent or low-stage CT findings are much less defined and controversial. Nonetheless, the authors' clinical protocol requires certain criteria be met before considering a potential rhinogenic source for the headache.

First, the region of the headache should be consistent anatomically with the paranasal sinus. This criterion includes facial pain limited to the frontalis, midface, retro-orbital, or occipital regions. Temporal and band-like headaches should not be considered, because these presentations are more consistently identifiable as tension-related or myofacial. Second, the headache or facial pain should be associated with either of the following conditions: (1) symptoms worsen with flight, diving, or change in weather; (2) symptoms improve when a topical nasal decongestants or anesthetic agent is administered; or (3) symptoms are consistently associated with congestion or rhinitis. Exclusionary symptoms include headaches with rhinitis or congestion that occur in the middle of the night, suggesting a cluster headache, or unilateral, pulsatile headaches that are more associated with migraine and migraine-variant headaches. Currently, an imaging criterion is not included, because no established hallmark or consistent radiographic abnormalities definitively identify a rhinogenic cause.

IMAGING

The following are radiographic case examples from a retrospective review of prior patients and a review of the literature reporting on patients who were diagnosed with a rhinogenic source of headache or facial pain. These subsets of patients have absent or minimal mucosal findings radiographically but have been diagnosed with a rhinogenic headache, and are often treated medically or procedurally based primarily on clinical presentation. Nonetheless, these patients have structural abnormalities seen on CT scans that are at least suggestive of a cause. These imaging variants include contact-point headaches that have representative mucosal contact areas within the nasal cavity, often from the septum to various lateral nasal wall structures.[11–19]

Also included are representative CT images from patients with RARS between active episodes. These case samples demonstrate various examples of outflow tract obstruction points, including narrowing of the infundibular space.

Table 1
Symptomatic criteria for potential rhinogenic headache

Inclusion Criteria	Exclusion Criteria
FP/HA limited to the frontalis, midface, retro-orbital, and occipital regions AND	FP/HA with rhinitis or congestion that occurs in the middle of the night (cluster headache)
FP/HA worsens with flight, diving, or change in weather OR	Unilateral, pulsatile headaches (migraine headaches)
FP/HA improves with application of a topical nasal decongestant or anesthetic agent OR	
FP/HA associated with congestion or rhinitis	

Abbreviations: FP, facial pain; HA, headache.

Septal Spur Abutting the Inferior Turbinate

A 49-year-old man treated for "sinus" problems with antibiotics and nasal sprays most of his life presented with persistent headaches. Topical 2% tetracaine with oxymetazoline placed between the spur and the inferior turbinate reduced the headache severity. The CT scan (**Fig. 1**) showed a prominent septal spur abutting the inferior turbinate, causing a potential mucosal contact-point.[11–15,19] The patient underwent a septoplasty that relieved his symptoms.

Septal Spur Abutting the Middle Turbinate

A patient presented with nasal obstruction and intermittent headaches associated with rhinitis. CT imaging showed a large bony septal spur abutting the middle turbinate (**Fig. 2**). After treatment with nasal corticosteroids failed, a septoplasty with turbinate reduction improved his persistent nasal obstruction and headaches.

Concha Bullosa of the Middle Turbinate

A 44-year-old patient presented with recurrent mid-facial headaches. CT scan (**Fig. 3**) revealed mucosal contact of the middle turbinate with the septum from a large obstructing concha bullosa. The patient underwent a septoplasty with reduction of the middle turbinate and concha bullosa, relieving his symptoms.

Concha Bullosa of the Superior Turbinate

An 83-year-old with a 5-year history of recurrent headaches involving the frontalis region presented with a potential contact point from his right superior turbinate to his septum secondary to a concha bullosa of the superior turbinate (**Fig 4**). An in-office reduction of the turbinate reduced the severity and frequency of his headaches.

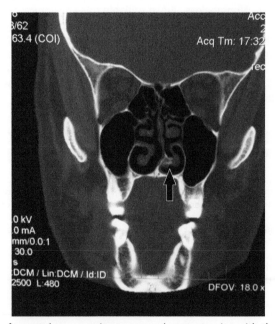

Fig. 1. CT image of a septal spur causing a mucosal contact point with the septum (*arrow*).

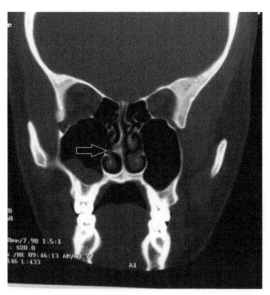

Fig. 2. CT scan showing a large bony septal spur that abuts the middle turbinate (*arrow*).

Haller Cell

A 29-year-old man with suspected RARS presented after being treated medically with multiple antibiotics and long-term nasal corticosteroids. Dull maxillary facial pain and headache were relieved with topical decongestants. A CT scan (**Fig. 5**) taken while he was asymptomatic revealed a Haller cell, or ethmoid cells that pneumatize laterally into the medial or inferior orbital wall above the maxillary ostium. Haller cells have

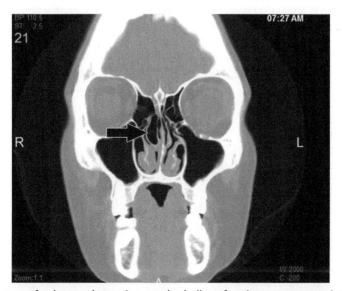

Fig. 3. CT scan of a large, obstructing concha bullosa forming a contact point with the septum (*arrow*).

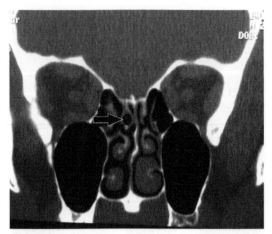

Fig. 4. CT image showing a superior turbinate concha bullosa (*arrow*) causing a mucosal contact point with the septum.

been associated with RARS.[5] In this case, the Haller cell may contribute to intermittent obstruction of the maxillary os.

Small Infundibular Widths

An 81-year-old woman who was diagnosed clinically with RARS presented with a primary complaint of recurrent left-sided facial pain. CT imaging (**Fig. 6**) showed a small infundibular width with an adjacent hypertrophic middle turbinate. Smaller infundibular widths (<0.591 mm) have been associated with RARS.[5] The concha bullosa on the opposite side is less consequential to her headaches.

Paradoxic Middle Turbinates

In a patient who originally presented with nasal obstruction, congestion, and associated headaches, a CT scan revealed paradoxic curvature of the right middle turbinate

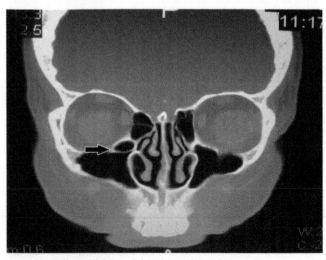

Fig. 5. CT image of a Haller cell (*arrow*) blocking the right maxillary sinus outflow tract.

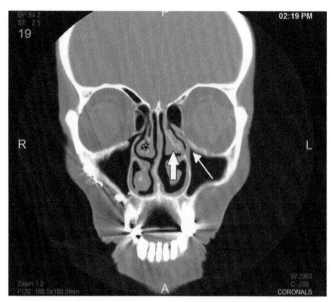

Fig. 6. CT image of a narrowed infundibular width (thin *white arrow*), adjacent obstructing middle turbinate (*thick white arrow*), and concha bullosa (*star*).

(**Fig. 7**). Paradoxic turbinates have also been shown to be a potential mucosal contact between the middle turbinate and the septum.[20,21]

Atelectatic Maxillary Sinus

A 38-year-old recently diagnosed with human immunodeficiency virus presented with intermittent right-sided facial pain. Purulent debris cultured from the right side

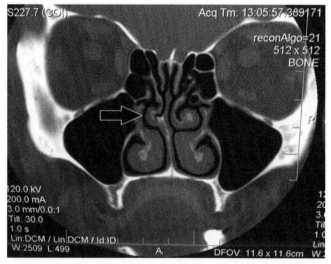

Fig. 7. CT scan of a right-sided paradoxic middle turbinate (*arrow*) adjacent to a septal bony spur.

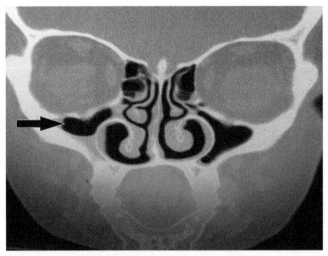

Fig. 8. CT image showing atelectatic maxillary sinuses (*arrow*).

osteomeatal complex grew *Propionibacterium* spp, *Curvularia* spp, and *Staphylococcus aureus*. After several rounds of antibiotics, the patient underwent a CT scan while asymptomatic, which revealed an atelectatic maxillary sinus suggestive of a recurrent infection (**Fig. 8**). Chronic maxillary sinusitis has been associated with atelectasis.[11,22–25]

SUMMARY

Rhinogenic headaches encompass a broad spectrum of potential causes that result in facial pain and headaches. From an imaging standpoint, outside of well-established diagnostic criteria of mucosal findings within the paranasal sinuses for acute/chronic sinusitis, diagnostic imaging criteria for rhinogenic headaches are challenging. Nonetheless, standard CT scans potentially identify structural abnormalities that may result in mucosal contact points or inhibit outflow tracts of the paranasal sinuses. These findings may be common variants, such as concha bullosas, septal spurs, Haller cells, paradoxic middle turbinates, and small infundibular widths. However, when coupled with clinical history, these findings may support a rhinogenic cause. Identifying these minor imaging variations allows for better identification of recalcitrant headaches. Consideration of these findings will also help in the surgical planning, specifically for rhinogenic headaches, and determining the potential for performing minimally invasive techniques.

REFERENCES

1. Rosenfeld RM. Clinical practice guideline on adult sinusitis. Otolaryngol Head Neck Surg 2007;137:65–77.
2. Rosenfeld RM, Andes D, Bhattacharyya N, et al. Clinical practice guideline: adult sinusitis. Otolaryngol Head Neck Surg 2007;137(Suppl 3):S1–31.
3. Levine HL, Setzen M, Cady RK, et al. An otolaryngology, neurology, allergy, and primary care consensus on diagnosis and treatment of sinus headache. Otolaryngol Head Neck Surg 2006;134:516–23.
4. Poetker DM, Litvack JR, Mace JC, et al. Recurrent acute rhinosinusitis: presentation and outcomes of sinus surgery. Am J Rhinol 2008;22(3):329–33.

5. Alkire BC, Bhattacharyya N. An assessment of sinonasal anatomic variants potentially associated with recurrent acute rhinosinusitis. Laryngoscope 2010; 120(3):631–4.
6. Leung R, Kern RC, Conley DB, et al. Establishing a threshold for surgery in recurrent acute rhinosinusitis: a productivity-based analysis. Otolaryngol Head Neck Surg 2012;146(5):829–33.
7. Meltzer EO, Hamilos DL. Rhinosinusitis diagnosis and management for the clinician: a synopsis of recent consensus guidelines. Mayo Clin Proc 2011;86(5): 427–43.
8. Yarmohammadi ME, Ghasemi H, Pourfarzam S, et al. Effect of turbinoplasty in concha bullosa induced rhinogenic headache, a randomized clinical trial. J Res Med Sci 2012;17(3):229–34.
9. Stewart TW Jr. Common otolarygologic problems of flying. Am Fam Physician 1979;19(2):113–9.
10. Rudmik L, Muzychuck A, Oddone Paolucci E, et al. Chinook wind barosinusitis: an anatomic evaluation. Am J Rhinol Allergy 2009;23(6):e14–6.
11. Boyd JH, Yaffee K, Holds J. Maxillary sinus atelectasis with enophthalmos. Ann Otol Rhinol Laryngol 1998;107(1):34–9.
12. Mariotti LJ, Setliff RC III, Ghaderi M, et al. Patient history and CT findings in predicting surgical outcomes for patients with rhinogenic headache. Ear Nose Throat J 2009;88:926–9.
13. Uygur K, Tuz M, Dogru H. The correlation between septal deviation and concha bullosa. Otolaryngol Head Neck Surg 2003;129:33–6.
14. Bolger WE, Butzin CA, Parsons DS. Paranasal sinus bony anatomic variations and mucosal abnormalities: CT analysis for endoscopic sinus surgery. Laryngoscope 1991;101:56–64.
15. Huang HH, Lee TJ, Huang CC, et al. Non-sinusitis-related rhinogenous headache: a ten-year experience. Am J Otolaryngol 2008;29:326–33.
16. Nselmo-Lima WT, de Oliveira JA, Speciali JG, et al. Middle turbinate headache syndrome. Headache 1997;37:102–6.
17. Peric A, Baletic N, Sotirovic J. A case of an uncommon anatomic variation of the middle turbinate associated with headache. Acta Otorhinolaryngol Ital 2010;30: 156–9.
18. Harrison L, Jones NS. Intranasal contact points as a cause of facial pain or headache. Clin Otolaryngol 2013;38:8–22.
19. Earwaker J. Anatomic variants in sinonasal CT. Radiographics 1993;13:381–415.
20. Roozbahany NA, Nasri S. Nasal and paranasal sinus anatomical variations in patients with rhinogenic contact point headache. Auris Nasus Larynx 2013;40: 177–83.
21. Perez-Pinas I, Sabate J, Carmona A. Anatomical variations in the human paranasal sinus regions studied by CT. J Anat 2000;197:221–7.
22. Virgin F, Ling FT, Kountakis SE. Radiology and endoscopic findings of silent maxillary sinus atelectasis and enophthalmos. Am J Otolaryngol 2008;29(3): 167–70.
23. Kohn JC, Rootman DB, Xu D, et al. Infratemporal fossa fat enlargement in chronic maxillary atelectasis. Br J Ophthalmol 2013;97(8):1005–9.
24. Annino DJ Jr, Goguen LA. Silent sinus syndrome. Curr Opin Otolaryngol Head Neck Surg 2008;16(1):22–5.
25. Wise SK, Wojno TH, DelGaudio JM. Silent sinus syndrome: lack of orbital findings in early presentation. Am J Rhinol 2007;21(4):489–94.

Imaging for Headache
What the Neuroradiologist Looks For

Aliye Bricker, MD*, Todd Stultz, MD, DDS

KEYWORDS

- Computed tomography • Magnetic resonance imaging • Sinusitis • Headache

KEY POINTS

- Computed tomography is the primary modality for imaging the paranasal sinuses, as it optimally delineates bony anatomy and can provide an accurate roadmap before surgery.
- Magnetic resonance imaging is superior in assessing the extent of involvement of intracranial, intraorbital, or deep fascial soft tissues in complicated cases.
- Basic knowledge of the primary sinus outflow tracts is crucial to understanding the pathology of sinus disease.
- Though relatively rare, aggressive infectious and neoplastic processes can occur within the paranasal sinuses, which may initially present with rhinogenic headache.

INTRODUCTION AND OVERVIEW

When patients referred to otolaryngologists with headaches of suspected rhinogenic or paranasal sinus–related origin are imaged, the neuroradiologist's job is to define anatomy, characterize any potential obstructive abnormality, screen for underlying neoplasm or destructive process, and evaluate for associated involvement of adjacent orbital, intracranial, and deep facial structures. Although radiographic imaging of the paranasal sinuses is generally not necessary for patients who meet clinical criteria for uncomplicated rhinosinusitis,[1] imaging proves useful in defining the anatomy of the sinuses before surgery and in aiding the management of chronic or recurrent rhinosinusitis.

BASIC IMAGING ANATOMY AND STANDARD IMAGING TECHNIQUES

Understanding the normal anatomic and physiologic outflow pathways of mucociliary clearance from the paranasal sinuses is essential to identifying and accurately

Division of Neuroradiology, Cleveland Clinic Foundation, 9500 Euclid Avenue, Cleveland, OH 44195, USA
* Corresponding author.
E-mail address: brickea2@ccf.org

Otolaryngol Clin N Am 47 (2014) 197–219
http://dx.doi.org/10.1016/j.otc.2013.10.009   oto.theclinics.com

Abbreviations	
CT	Computed tomography
MRI	Magnetic resonance imaging
OMC	Osteomeatal complex
FESS	Functional endoscopic sinus surgery

delineating the pathogenesis of rhinosinusitis, and ultimately to restoring physiologic drainage patterns via functional endoscopic sinus surgery (FESS). Key to this are the frontal recess, sphenoethmoid recess, and the ostiomeatal complex (OMC), which refers to the maxillary sinus ostium, the infundibulum, the uncinate process, hiatus semilunaris, the ethmoid bulla, and the middle meatus. Together, the components of the OMC provide the common drainage pathway of the frontal sinuses, maxillary sinuses, and anterior ethmoid air cells.

Drainage from the maxillary sinuses is directed superomedially toward the maxillary infundibulum, located lateral to the uncinate process and inferomedial to the orbit, through the hiatus semilunaris and posteromedially through the middle meatus to the back of the nasal cavity and into the nasopharynx. There is a strong correlation between opacification of the osteomeatal complex and the presence or development of sinusitis, with inflammatory changes of the maxillary sinuses seen in approximately 80% of patients with infundibular opacification and in 82% of patients with middle meatus opacification.[2]

The frontal sinuses and anterior ethmoid air cells drain inferomedially via the frontal recess (or frontoethmoidal recess) down to the middle meatus. The posterior ethmoid air cells are located behind the basal lamella or lateral attachment of the middle nasal turbinate to the lamina papyracea of the orbit. Drainage from the posterior ethmoid air cells and sphenoid sinuses is via the sphenoethmoidal recess down into the nasopharynx. These key structures and the major anatomic outflow tracts are illustrated in **Fig. 1**.

When imaging the paranasal sinuses, computed tomography (CT) without intravenous contrast is the imaging modality of choice. CT provides optimal delineation of osseous anatomy and, using multidetector helical CT acquisition techniques, can acquire thin, high-resolution axial scans with 0.75-mm collimation and 1-mm slice thickness with sagittal, coronal, or oblique reconstructions in less than a minute. These shorter scan times help limit motion artifact, reduce radiation exposure, and make CT more tolerable for patients who have difficulty lying prone or supine. Given the substantially different density of the aerated sinus, dense osseous margins of the paranasal sinus chambers and lower-density fat-containing tissues of the adjacent orbits, iodinated intravenous contrast is generally not necessary for most routine examinations. However, in cases of suspected early subperiosteal abscess or orbital involvement, contrast-enhanced images can better define small, peripherally enhancing abscess collections or extent of orbital involvement. Renal dysfunction is a relative contraindication to administering intravenous contrast, and should be avoided if the glomerular filtration rate (GFR) is less than 30.

Although magnetic resonance imaging (MRI) is limited with regard to bony detail, for those patients in whom neoplasm is suspected, or when there is need to further define the extent of orbital or intracranial involvement, MRI provides superior definition of the mucosa, adjacent soft tissues, and brain parenchyma. Particularly when osseous dehiscence is identified along the frontal, sphenoid, or ethmoid paranasal sinuses in a patient with altered mental status and sinusitis, MRI is essential to evaluate for

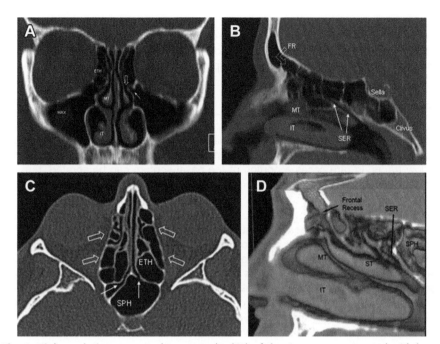

Fig. 1. High-resolution computed tomography (CT) of the sinuses reconstructed with bone algorithm. (*A*) Coronal view best demonstrating the osteomeatal complexes and components: maxillary infundibulum (*arrow*), uncinate process, and overlying hiatus semilunaris (*open arrow*) with adjacent middle meatus just medially. Middle (MT) and inferior nasal turbinates (IT), maxillary sinuses (MAX), and ethmoid air cells (ETH) are also shown. (*B*) Midline sagittal reconstruction demonstrating frontal sinuses frontal recess (FR, *open arrow*) draining the frontal sinuses and anterior ethmoid air cells, and the sphenoethmoidal recess (SER, *arrows*) draining the sphenoid sinuses and posterior ethmoid air cells down into the nasopharynx. Sphenoid ostia are not included on this image. Clivus, floor of the anterior cranial fossa, and sella are also seen. (*C*) Axial view through the sphenoid ostia (*arrows*) opening into the sphenoethmoidal recesses, sphenoid sinuses (SPH), and ethmoid air cells (ETH), bound laterally by a thin rim of bone known as the lamina papyracea, which also serves as the medial orbital wall (*open arrows*). (*D*) Three-dimensional rendered sagittal CT image demonstrating the frontal recess (*arrow*), and sphenoethmoidal recess (SER) draining the sphenoid sinuses (SPH). Superior nasal turbinate (ST), middle nasal turbinate (MT), and inferior nasal turbinate (IT) are also shown.

findings of secondary subdural empyema or intracranial abscess, which may not be as apparent on CT alone. Sinonasal secretions and areas of mucosal thickening will demonstrate varied signal characteristics on MRI depending on protein content, thereby providing additional insight into chronicity of inflammation (see later discussion). Major limitations of MRI are increased cost and longer scan times, which can prove difficult for patients who are in discomfort and unable to keep still. Certain patients with non–MRI-compatible implanted devices are also unable to safely undergo MRI.

ANATOMIC VARIANTS THAT MAY PREDISPOSE TO RHINOGENIC HEADACHE

Any anatomic variant that obstructs 1 or more of the 3 major sinus outflow tracts can potentially predispose to obstructive sinus inflammation. The most common of these are discussed here. As CT now frequently serves as a roadmap for surgeons before functional endoscopic surgery, identification of certain specific anatomic variants, such as localized osseous dehiscence along the osseous margins of the posterior ethmoid or sphenoid sinuses underlying the optic nerves, nasofrontal, nasoethmoidal, and nasoorbital encephaloceles, is of utmost importance preoperatively to prevent potentially devastating intraoperative complications such as inadvertent orbital or intracranial entry.

Septal Variants

The nasal septum is the midline structure separating the right and left superior, middle, and inferior nasal turbinates. Bowing or deviation of the nasal septum is very common, often with bony spurring at the apex of deviation, which may compromise the OMC outflow tracts. In rare cases a portion of the nasal septum can be aerated, termed septum bullosa.

Concha Bullosa

When one or both of the nasal turbinates is aerated, this is termed a concha bullosa (**Fig. 2**). Concha bullosa most commonly occur within the middle nasal turbinates, seen in approximately 34% to 53% of patients, with significant pneumatization of the inferior or superior nasal turbinates seen in fewer than 10%.[2] When large enough, concha bullosa may obstruct the middle meatus, maxillary infundibulum, or any number of sinus outflow pathways. The mucous membrane lining the concha bullosa is no different from the rest of the sinuses and may also display inflammatory changes, including development of fluid-fluid levels.

Uncinate Variants

The free edge of the uncinate process has a variable course. Lateral deviation narrows the infundibulum. Medial deviation may narrow or obstruct the middle meatus. Occasionally, the free edge of the uncinate is fused to the orbital floor or lamina papyracea, described as an atelectatic uncinate process. Inflammation or hypoplasia of the ipsilateral maxillary sinus may be present, related to partial or complete obstruction of the infundibulum. Occasionally the uncinate may be aerated.

Ethmoid Variants

Ethmoid air cells extending along the inferior margin of the orbit are termed Haller cells (**Fig. 3**), which are seen in 10% to 45% of patients.[2] When large enough, Haller cells can cause narrowing or obstruction of the infundibulum. The anteriormost ethmoid

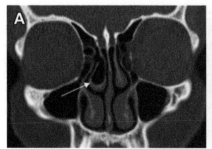 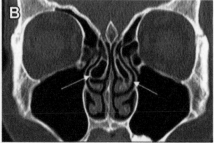

Fig. 2. Coronal CT images from 2 different patients demonstrating concha bullosa of the right middle nasal turbinate (*arrow in A*) and of both middle nasal turbinates (*arrows in B*). This developmental variant does not appear to cause significant obstruction of the osteomeatal complex in either of these two patients, both of whom have clear sinuses.

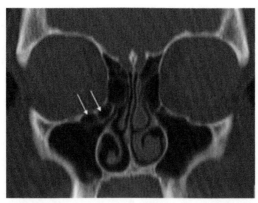

Fig. 3. Coronal CT image demonstrating right-sided Haller cells (*arrows*). Although the adjacent right maxillary infundibulum remains patent, in the presence of inflammation this developmental variant might predispose to obstruction of the right maxillary sinus.

air cells are termed agger nasi cells, which are immediately anterior and inferior to the frontal recess, and can thus narrow or potentially obstruct drainage from the frontal sinuses if large enough. Agger nasi cells are also in close proximity to the nasolacrimal ducts as they course inferiorly from the medial canthus, and can be a source of epiphora when inflammatory changes are present. Onodi cells are rare, posteriormost ethmoid air cells overlying the sphenoid sinuses, which are important to note given their close proximity to the optic nerves.

Rhinogenic Headache in the Absence of Sinusitis

In 1948, Wolff[3] demonstrated that traction on different regions of the meninges and stimulation of various areas in the sinuses produced facial pain and headache. Over the past several decades, numerous studies have documented overall subjective improvement of headaches and facial pain following surgery directed at various contact points between 2 opposing mucosal surfaces within the nasal cavities,[4,5] most commonly occurring between an osseous spur along a deviated nasal septum and the adjacent middle or nasal turbinate, or between a large concha bullosa and the uncinate process or lateral nasal wall. Certain patients with refractory headaches who have failed medical treatment directed at migraine and have no signs of underlying sinonasal inflammatory change, but demonstrate contact points on CT or endoscopy, may thus benefit from directed nasal surgery.[6] Although mucosal contact points may be present in normal, asymptomatic patients who are scanned for other reasons, these anatomic variants can be another potential cause for rhinogenic headache, and are thus important to identify (**Fig. 4**).

INFECTIOUS OR INFLAMMATORY
Findings of Acute Versus Chronic Sinusitis

CT findings do not always correlate with severity of suspected rhinogenic or sinus-related symptoms, with incidental mucosal thickening noted on the CT scans of asymptomatic patients in as many as 5% to 40% of cases.[7–9] Furthermore, the location of mucosal thickening within the paranasal sinuses may be more important than the extent. In other words, a subtle area of opacification within the infundibulum,

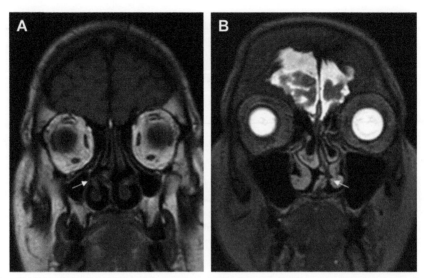

Fig. 4. (*A*). Coronal T1-weighted image from MRI of the brain performed in a young patient with headaches demonstrating rightward nasal septal deviation and spur formation, which contacts the right inferior nasal turbinate (*arrow*). The brain was normal in appearance. (*B*) Coronal T2-weighted MR image of a patient without headaches or rhinogenic symptoms, demonstrating leftward nasal septal deviation with contact of left inferior nasal turbinate (*arrow*). There are also nonobstructing concha bullosa of the middle nasal turbinates bilaterally.

sphenoethmoidal, or frontal recess may cause more discomfort for the patient than near complete opacification of the maxillary sinus with a mucous retention cyst or polyp.[2] Nonetheless, CT imaging without intravenous contrast can establish the presence of inflammation in the paranasal sinuses,[1,10] and thereby provides an objective means of monitoring the extent of disease.

The mucosal surface of the normal paranasal sinus approximates the bone so closely that it is not visualized on CT, thus any soft-tissue attenuation seen along

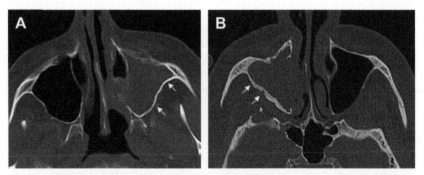

Fig. 5. Two different patients with chronic, complete obstruction of the maxillary sinus. Associated chronic inflammatory sclerosis and osseous thickening of the left maxillary sinus chamber walls are relatively mild in *A* (*arrows*), with more striking osseous thickening and sclerosis of the obstructed right maxillary sinus chamber walls in *B* (*arrows*), suggesting chronic inflammatory changes that have been present for a greater length of time.

the mucoperiosteal surfaces of the paranasal sinuses is abnormal. The presence of air-fluid levels has traditionally been associated with acute sinusitis, although the mere presence of fluid within the sinuses does not prove infection. Fluid from diagnostic or therapeutic lavage may remain for up to 2 weeks, and changes following a bout of acute sinusitis, even with successful therapy, may be seen for up to 6 to 8 weeks. In addition, acute sinusitis may be superimposed on chronic changes. Circumferential mucosal thickening without air-fluid level is nonspecific and can be seen in both the acute and chronic settings.

Classic findings of chronic sinusitis include polyposis, bony remodeling and thickening, and sclerosis related to osteitis from adjacent chronic mucosal inflammation (**Fig. 5**). As sinonasal secretions become chronically entrapped and the mucosa resorbs free water, the initially thin serous secretions transition to a thicker mucus with higher protein content, eventually forming a desiccated plug. Thinner secretions with higher water content will be hypodense on CT, whereas more viscous secretions with higher protein content will have gradually higher densities. This transition is even more strikingly apparent on MRI, where initially serous secretions with high water content will be T1-hypointense and T2-hyperintense; then, as protein concentration increases within the trapped, inspissated secretions, the T1 signal will increase while the T2 signal decreases (**Figs. 6** and **7**). As free water content further diminishes, the desiccated mucous plug will ultimately appear hypointense

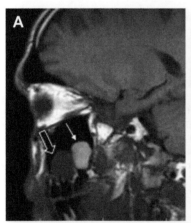
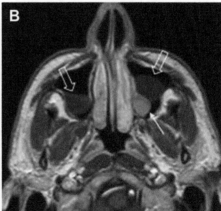
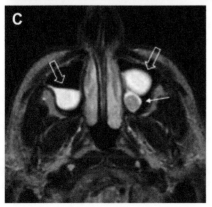

Fig. 6. Sagittal T1-weighted MR image (A), axial T1-weighted image (B), and axial T2-weighted image (C). Posterior focus of mucosal thickening within the left maxillary sinus shows T1-bright, T2-dark signal (*white arrows*) typical of more proteinaceous inspissated material and suggesting chronicity. Areas of mucosal thickening within the right and anterior left maxillary sinuses show signal typical of more serous secretion, with T1-dark and T2-bright signal (*open arrows*).

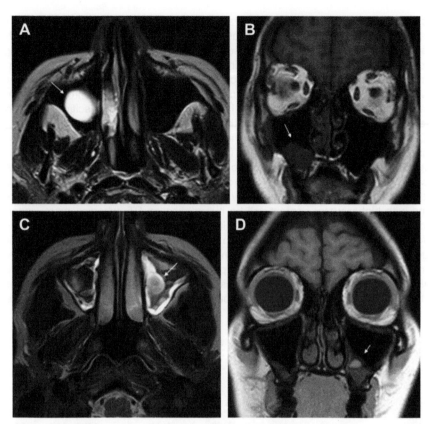

Fig. 7. Axial T2-weighted image (*A*) and Coronal T1-weighted image (*B*) demonstrating a simple mucous retention cyst within the right inferior maxillary sinus, which shows high T2 signal (*arrow in A*) and low T1 signal (*arrow in B*) compatible with more serous, high water content. Axial T2-weighted image (*C*) and coronal T1-weighted image (*D*) from a different patient demonstrating more extensive mucosal thickening of the maxillary sinuses bilaterally with left inferior maxillary mucous retention cyst demonstrating relatively lower T2 signal (*arrow in C*) with corresponding higher T1 signal (*arrow in D*) compatible with more chronic, inspissated secretions and higher protein content.

on both T1-weighted and T2-weighted images, nearly mimicking the normal aerated sinus.

Mucous Retention Cyst

Retention cysts are small, rounded, and smoothly circumscribed homogeneous, low-attenuation lesions, which generally occur along the floor of the maxillary sinuses of patients with a history of prior inflammation, thought to develop secondary to obstruction of small seromucinous glands within the sinus.[2,11] On MRI, more serous mucous retention cysts will demonstrate T1-dark, T2-bright signal following that of simple water, whereas more long-standing mucous retention cysts with increase in protein-aceous content will demonstrate a progressive increase in T1 signal with concomitant decrease in T2 signal (see **Fig. 7**). By imaging alone it is generally difficult to distinguish between a mucosal polyp or mucous retention cyst; however, this distinction is usually not of clinical significance unless the retention cyst is obstructive in size. In a review of 410 sinus CT scans to assess the clinical significance of maxillary sinus retention cysts, Bhattacharyya[12] demonstrated that maxillary sinus retention cysts are not associated with potentially obstructive anatomic variations, and do not reflect persistent obstructive abnormality.

Odontogenic Sinusitis

Pain related to odontogenic or periodontal disease can be easily mistakenly attributed to the sinuses. Given the close approximation of the maxillary premolar and molar roots to the floor of the maxillary sinuses, odontogenic sinus abnormality is a unique cause of infectious or inflammatory sinusitis that is typically limited to the maxillary sinuses. Advanced periodontal disease with overlying bony defects can serve as a nidus for persistent infection within the overlying maxillary sinus mucosa; however, perforated odontogenic cysts, failed endodontic therapy, or misplaced dental implants can also serve as additional potential causes of persistent inflammatory change within the overlying maxillary sinuses (**Fig. 8**).

Polyps and Polyposis

Inflammatory sinonasal polyposis most commonly occurs in the setting of allergic sinusitis, although isolated polyps may also occur secondary to localized mucosal hyperplasia from chronic inflammation. Even a solitary mucosal polyp can lead to significant postobstructive inflammatory change when located along one of the major sinonasal drainage pathways (**Fig. 9**). On CT and MRI, polyps are often indistinguishable from mucous retention cysts, both demonstrating hypoattenuation on CT and T1-dark, T2-bright signal on MRI; however, when present, identifying a thin, peduncular attachment point can be helpful in distinguishing a nasal polyp (**Fig. 10**). When large or numerous enough, polyps are associated with widening

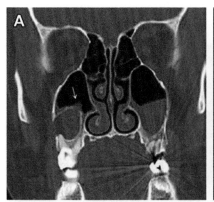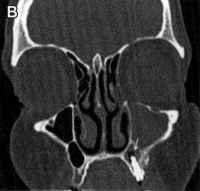

Fig. 8. Two coronal CT images from 2 different patients demonstrating an odontogenic cyst with perforation through the floor of the right maxillary sinus (*arrow in A*), and a root formed dental implant extending through the floor of the left maxillary sinus (*arrow in B*). Although the tip of these dental implants may often extend through the floor of the maxillary sinus, in this case there is air surrounding the tip of the implant and associated complete opacification with marked inflammatory changes of the overlying left maxillary sinus, suggesting odontogenic sinusitis.

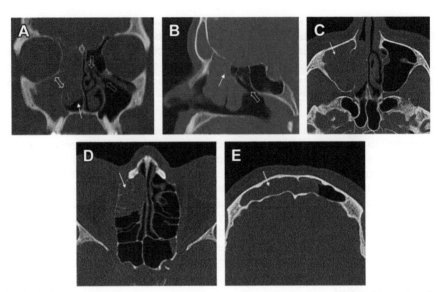

Fig. 9. Solitary nasal polyp centered within the right middle meatus and right nasal cavity (*white arrow,* coronal CT image *A*) results in obstruction of the right osteomeatal complex. There is obstruction and widening of the right maxillary infundibulum (*open 2-way arrow,* coronal CT image *A*) with additional obstruction of outflow from the right frontal recess (*white arrow,* sagittal CT image *B*). Subsequently there is complete, postobstructive opacification of the right maxillary sinus (axial CT image *C*), and also of the overlying right anterior ethmoid air cells (axial CT image *D*) and right frontal sinus (axial CT image *E*). Note that the left maxillary infundibulum and osteomeatal complex (*open dashed arrows in A*) remain open, and thus the left maxillary, left anterior ethmoid air cells and left frontal sinuses are clear. Because the sphenoethmoidal recess remains open (*open arrow in B*), the posterior ethmoid air cells and sphenoid sinuses are also essentially clear.

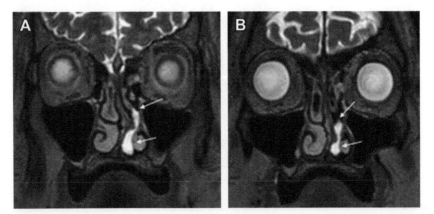

Fig. 10. (*A, B*) Coronal T2-weighted images demonstrating a T2-hyperintense nasal polyp extending inferiorly from the left middle nasal turbinate (*arrows*). Though infrequently visualized, identifying the thin, peduncular attachment helps distinguish nasal polyps from retained secretions.

of the infundibula or sphenoethmoidal recesses, and thinning of bony trabeculae (**Fig. 11**).

Mucocele

In cases of chronic ostial outflow obstruction, the osseous margins of the obstructed paranasal sinus chamber may undergo marked thinning and expansile remodeling to eventually form a mucocele (**Fig. 12**). CT best delineates the osseous margins of a mucocele, whereas MR signal characteristics may vary considerably because of the protein content. Interface between the mucocele and adjacent brain and/or orbital structures is best seen with MRI. Approximately 65% of mucoceles occur within the frontal sinuses, with ethmoid (25%), maxillary (10%), and sphenoid sinus mucoceles seen in decreasing order of frequency.[2,11] An infected mucocele is termed a muco-pyocele and may demonstrate a pattern of rim enhancement on contrast-enhanced MRI or CT, useful for distinguishing this expansile inflammatory condition from other slow-growing expansile sinonasal mass lesions such as an inverted papilloma, which demonstrate more solid enhancement.

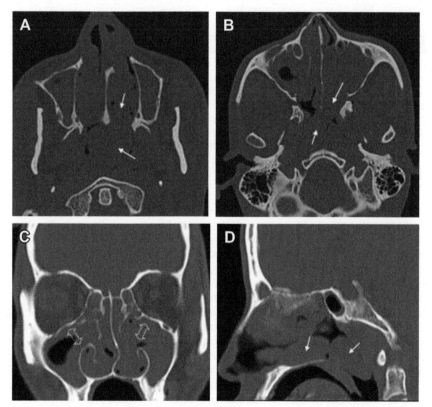

Fig. 11. Axial (*A*, *B*), coronal (*C*), and sagittal (*D*) CT images from a patient with nasal polyposis and pansinusitis, demonstrating characteristic ovoid and rounded lesions nearly completely opacifying the nasal cavities bilaterally, with widening of the infundibula (*open 2-way arrows*) and large soft tissue polyp extending into the nasopharynx (*white arrows*).

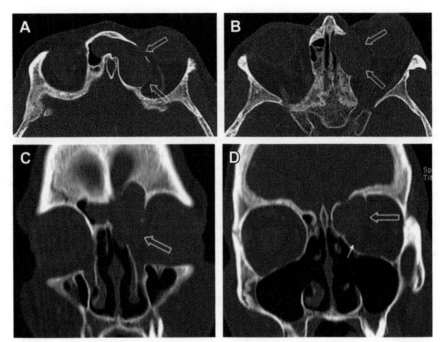

Fig. 12. Two axial (*A, B*) and 2 coronal (*C, D*) CT images from a patient with a left frontoethmoidal mucocele (*open arrows*) demonstrating characteristic expansile thinning and remodeling of the osseous sinus chamber walls, which are nearly imperceptible in several places. There is extension into the left medial, extraconal orbit (*open arrows in B and D*) with inferior displacement of the left medial rectus muscle (*white arrow in D*). This patient presented with visual disturbance and is incidentally also status post prior FESS, with resection of the uncinate processes and middle nasal turbinates bilaterally.

Fungal Infection

Fungal sinusitis can occur in both the immunocompetent and the immunocompromised host, and can manifest with differing levels of aggressiveness depending on the underlying pathogen. With aggressive, fulminant fungal sinusitis or in the immunocompromised patient, MRI is superior in evaluating for intracranial extension, involvement of the neurovascular structures, or associated vascular insults such as cavernous sinus thrombosis or cerebral infarcts. Fungal sinusitis, and specifically allergic fungal sinusitis, typically shows hyperdense secretions on CT manifesting as areas of punctuate hyperattenuation as seen in **Fig. 13**, or homogeneous hyperattenuation as shown in **Fig. 14**. However, it must be noted that markedly inspissated secretions hemorrhage into the sinus, and calcified masses will also appear hyperdense. MRI findings characteristic of fungal sinusitis are prominent dark signal on both T1-weighted and T2-weighted images, nearly mimicking that of the normally aerated sinus. Secretions with high protein content will demonstrate a characteristic T1-bright, T2-dark signal as previously discussed. Expansion, erosion, or expansile remodeling of the sinus chamber margins suggesting chronicity can be appreciated with both MRI and CT (see **Fig. 14**).

Granulomatous Infection

Granulomatous inflammatory changes of the sinuses may be infectious or noninfectious, with numerous potential underlying causes including actinomycosis,

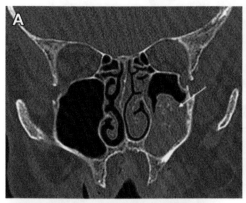

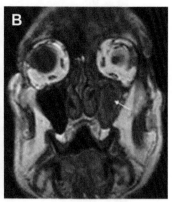

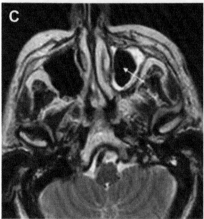

Fig. 13. CT and MR images of a patient with left maxillary fungal sinusitis, demonstrating characteristic punctate areas of hyperattenuation on CT (*arrow,* coronal CT image *A*) with heterogeneously dark T1 signal (*arrow,* coronal T1-weighted image *B*) and prominent signal drop-out on axial T2-weighted images (*arrow,* axial T2-weighted image *C*), which nearly mimics that of the normally aerated right maxillary sinus.

blastomycosis, leprosy, rhinoscleroma, syphilis, tuberculosis, sarcoidosis, and Wegener granulomatosis. Exuberant granulomatous response to certain foreign bodies in the setting of cocaine abuse or recurrent exposure to beryllium or chromate salts can also have a similar appearance. On imaging, these entities manifest with destruction of the cartilaginous, then the osseous midline nasal septum, with associated chronic inflammatory hypertrophic changes of the mucosa and osseous sinus chamber walls (**Fig. 15**).

Intracranial and Orbital Complications

Though rare, intracranial complications of rhinosinusitis can be devastating, estimated to be lethal in approximately 10% and permanently disabling in approximately 25% of affected individuals.[13] The most common intracranial complications of infectious rhinosinusitis are subdural empyema, intracranial abscess, meningitis, and intracranial thrombophlebitis. Infection most commonly spreads intracranially via the frontal, posterior ethmoid, and sphenoid sinuses, of which isolated sphenoiditis may present with the sole complaint of headache, without associated rhinologic symptoms.[13] Findings suggesting intracranial involvement can be very subtle on CT, which may demonstrate small areas of osseous dehiscence or fraying along the cribriform plate or fovea ethmoidalis, dorsal margins of the sphenoid sinuses, or ventral margins of the anterior cranial fossa. MRI with contrast best delineates the extent of associated subdural

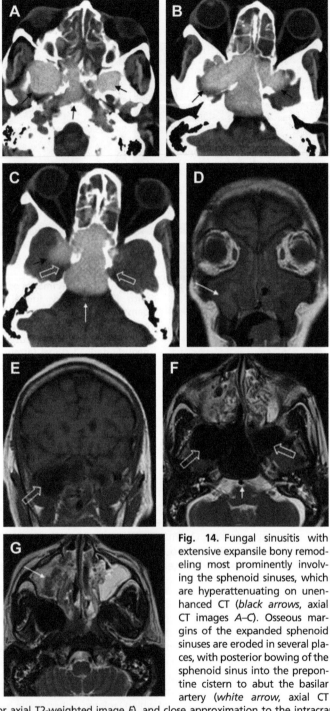

Fig. 14. Fungal sinusitis with extensive expansile bony remodeling most prominently involving the sphenoid sinuses, which are hyperattenuating on unenhanced CT (*black arrows*, axial CT images *A–C*). Osseous margins of the expanded sphenoid sinuses are eroded in several places, with posterior bowing of the sphenoid sinus into the prepontine cistern to abut the basilar artery (*white arrow*, axial CT image *C* or axial T2-weighted image *F*), and close approximation to the intracranial internal carotid arteries bilaterally (*open arrow*, axial CT image *C*). Hyperattenuating material throughout the expanded sphenoid sinuses demonstrates corresponding dark signal on both T1-weighted and T2-weighted MR images (*open arrows*, coronal T1-weighted image *E* and axial T2-weighted image *F*). Note varied T1 and T2 signal characteristics of secretions throughout both maxillary sinuses, with areas of increased T1 and decreased T2 signal reflecting material with higher protein content (*arrows*, coronal T1-weighted image *D* and axial T2-weighted image *G*).

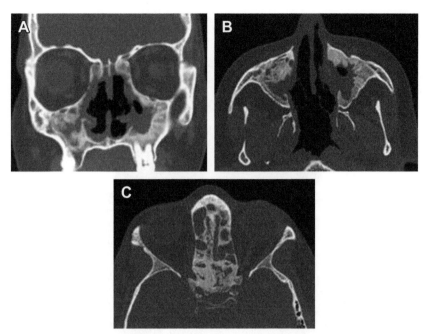

Fig. 15. Coronal (*A*) and axial (*B, C*) CT images of the paranasal sinuses in a patient with Wegener granulomatosis demonstrates destruction of the nasal septum with near complete opacification and prominent diffuse hypertrophic chronic inflammatory changes of the sinus chamber walls.

empyema (**Fig. 16**), intracranial abscess (**Fig. 17**), edema of the adjacent brain parenchyma suggesting associated cerebritis, or diffuse leptomeningeal enhancement that can be seen in the setting of meningitis.

Orbital involvement is another feared complication of acute sinusitis, ranging from simple preseptal (in front of the orbit) soft-tissue swelling and cellulitis (see **Fig. 17**) to postseptal (posterior to the orbit) inflammation with subperiosteal or intraorbital abscess requiring emergent surgical evaluation (**Fig. 18**). These complications most frequently occur secondary to spread of infection from the ethmoid air cells into the adjacent medial orbit through the very thin rim of bone separating the two, known as the lamina papyracea. Tiny anatomic foci of osseous dehiscence along the lamina papyracea (known as dehiscence of Zuckerkandl) can also serve as a direct means for spread of infection into the adjacent orbit. Although intraorbital complications of sinusitis are more common in the pediatric population, spread of infection beyond the sinuses can occur in any patient based on their immune status or the underlying pathogen. When intraorbital involvement is suspected, CT with intravenous contrast is best for initial evaluation given the speed with which images can be obtained in the emergent setting, and optimal delineation of surgical anatomy. Findings of subperiosteal abscess include a crescentic or ovoid collection of peripherally enhancing, centrally hypoattenuating fluid, which may occasionally also contain gas (see **Fig. 18**) most commonly seen within the medial, extraconal orbit and along the lamina papyracea overlying adjacent ethmoidal inflammatory change. Though less common, direct spread of infection can also occur into the inferior orbit from the adjacent maxillary sinuses, or into the superior orbit from the adjacent frontal sinuses. In rare cases where orbital involvement is highly suspected clinically but not appreciable on CT,

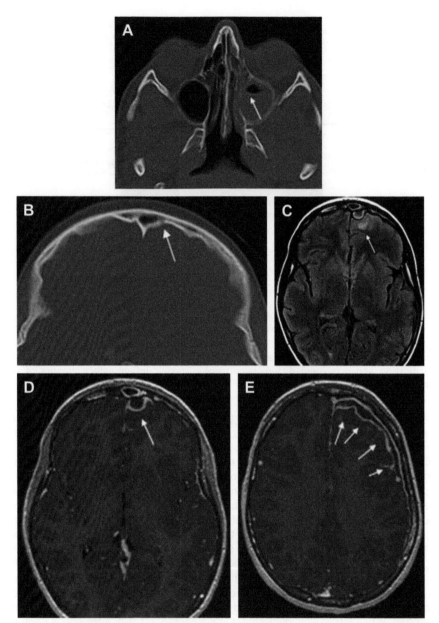

Fig. 16. Young patient with headache, sinonasal congestion, and altered mental status. Axial CT images demonstrate opacification of the left maxillary sinus (*A*), anterior ethmoid air cells and left frontal sinus with air-fluid level within left maxillary sinus, suggesting component of acuity (*arrow in A*). Tiny focus of osseous dehiscence along the posterior left frontal sinus is subtle on CT (*arrow,* axial CT image *B*), although associated left frontal subdural empyema with edema of the adjacent brain parenchyma is well delineated on subsequent fluid-attenuated inversion recovery (FLAIR) (*arrow in C*) and contrast-enhanced T1-weighted MR images (*arrows in D, E*).

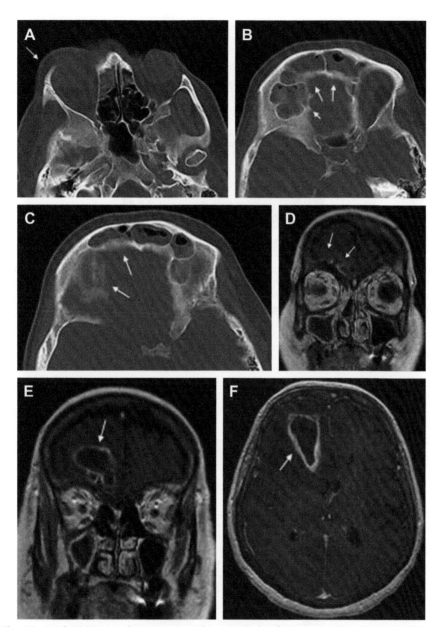

Fig. 17. Axial CT images demonstrate right preseptal soft-tissue swelling (*arrow in A*), in-flammatory changes of the frontal sinuses, and somewhat frayed appearance of the osseous margins of the right frontal sinus and cribriform plate (*arrows in B, C*), concerning for intra-cranial involvement. Subsequent MRI demonstrates meningeal enhancement along right anterior cranial fossa (*arrows*, coronal postcontrast T1-weighted image *D*) with large rim-enhancing abscess collection (*arrows*, postcontrast T1-weighted images *E, F*).

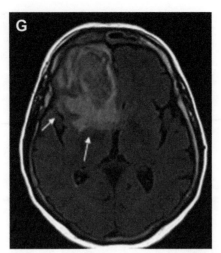

Fig. 17. (*continued*) Osseous margins of the right frontal sinus and cribriform plate concerning for intracranial involvement. MRI demonstrates extensive surrounding edema manifesting as FLAIR hyperintense signal within the overlying right anterior frontal lobe with associated effacement of sulci (*arrows*, axial FLAIR image *G*).

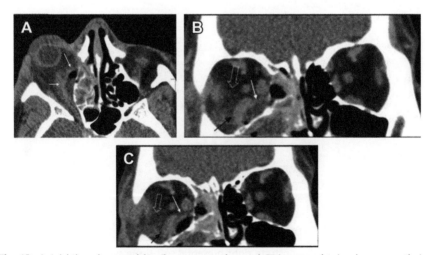

Fig. 18. Axial (*A*) and coronal (*B, C*) contrast-enhanced CT images obtained emergently in a patient with symptoms of sinusitis and progressive proptosis. Abnormal centrally hypoattenuating, rim-enhancing fluid collection containing small amounts of air and compatible with abscess (*arrows*) seen within the inferomedial, extraconal orbit overlying the right lamina papyracea and roof of the right maxillary sinus, likely secondary to direct spread of infection from the adjacent right maxillary sinus and ethmoid air cells that demonstrate marked inflammatory change with near complete opacification. There is superomedial displacement of the right inferior rectus muscle (*black arrow in B, C*). Note the asymmetric haziness of the retroorbital fat (*open arrows*) within the right inferior orbit, compatible with associated inflammation.

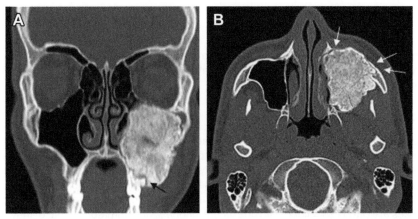

Fig. 19. Large osteoma of the maxillary sinus. This young patient presented with slowly progressive facial asymmetry and toothaches. CT best delineates the large mass arising from the maxilla with osseous mineralization following that of the adjacent bone. Findings suggesting chronicity and relatively slow-growing process include well-defined sclerotic margins, remodeling of the underlying teeth without destruction (*arrow in A*), and expansile remodeling of the overlying maxillary sinus walls (*arrows in B*). Osteomas are one of the most common osseous lesions of the paranasal sinuses, and often occur in the frontal sinuses. When large enough to obstruct one of the sinonasal outflow tracts, these benign lesions can cause headache, postobstructive sinusitis, or mucocele formation.

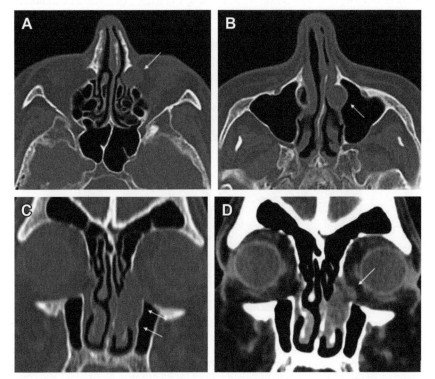

Fig. 20. Low-grade myoepithelial carcinoma of the nasolacrimal duct. This patient presented with headaches, chronic and progressive epiphora, and tearing of the left eye. Axial CT images (*A, B*) demonstrate smoothly marginated, expansile thinning of the osseous margins of the nasolacrimal duct (*arrows*), suggesting a long-standing process. Coronal CT images in bone (*C*) and soft-tissue (*D*) windows demonstrate the extent of the soft-tissue mass extending from the level of the inferior turbinate up to the inferomedial orbit.

contrast-enhanced MRI of the orbits using fat saturation and dedicated small-field-of-view images can reveal intraorbital complications that may be obscured or simply not evident on CT.[14]

NASAL AND PARANASAL MASSES

Masses arising within the nasal cavity and paranasal sinuses constitute only 3% to 4% of all head and neck neoplasms,[15] but comprise a wide spectrum of pathologic features secondary to the numerous different types of tissue that make up the complex anatomy of these structures, including osseous, cartilaginous, minor salivary gland tissue, and squamous epithelium. Because masses of the nasal cavity and paranasal sinuses are often associated with coexistent sinonasal inflammatory disease, they are often overlooked by the patient and the clinician until they have either grown very large or are associated with significant pain from invasion of adjacent structures such as the skull base, orbit, or infratemporal fossa. Although a detailed discussion of each of these pathologic conditions is beyond the scope of this article, it is important to be able to differentiate between high-grade, destructive neoplasms associated with adjacent orbital or intracranial extension and more slow-growing, relatively nonaggressive lesions. Examples of each are provided here. CT and MRI have complementary roles in the assessment and staging of these neoplasms, with CT superior in delineating osseous structures and MRI better for evaluating the extent of invasion into adjacent brain, orbit, or soft-tissue structures.

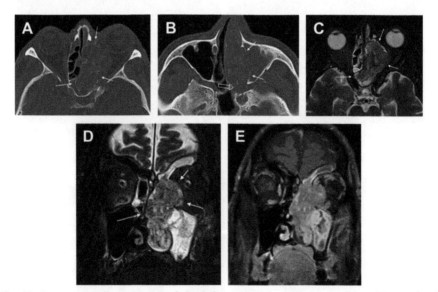

Fig. 21. Squamous cell carcinoma of the left nasal cavity with paranasal and intraorbital involvement. Axial CT images best demonstrate osseous destruction of the ethmoid septa, margins of the sphenoid sinus, and left lamina papyracea (*arrows in A*). as well as osseous destruction of the medial left maxillary sinus and left nasolacrimal duct (*arrows in B*) and extension posteriorly into left pterygopalatine fossa (*open arrow in B*). Axial (*C*) and coronal (*D*) T2-weighted MR images demonstrate characteristic T2-dark signal associated with the mass, which extends into the left medial orbit (*arrows*). Note how the T2-dark signal of cellular neoplasm contrasts with the T2-bright signal of retained secretions within the contralateral right-sided ethmoid air cells. Mass demonstrates heterogeneous enhancement on contrast-enhanced coronal T1-weighted image (*E*).

Features that suggest a slow-growing and, therefore, relatively benign process include smooth thinning or expansile remodeling of adjacent osseous structures and/or displacement of adjacent structures without frank destruction (**Figs. 19 and 20**). Though less specific, well-defined margins can suggest a less infiltrative, more localized mass. Likewise, lack of enhancement also suggests relatively less vascularized mass. Examples of benign neoplasms occurring within the nasal cavities and paranasal sinuses include osteomas, fibrous dysplasia, enchondromas, papillomas, extradural meningiomas, and many others.

Aggressive masses of the nasal cavity or paranasal sinuses are characterized by localized destruction of adjacent structures, initially best demonstrated on CT either by complete osseous obliteration or by more subtle erosion of the skull-base foramina. To determine the best course of therapy for these patients, great care must be taken to accurately delineate the degree of contiguous extension into the adjacent orbit and overlying anterior or middle cranial fossa, or the presence of perineural spread, for which MRI is the imaging modality of choice. Squamous cell carcinoma accounts for 80% of sinonasal malignancies, with 30% of these arising within the nasal cavity

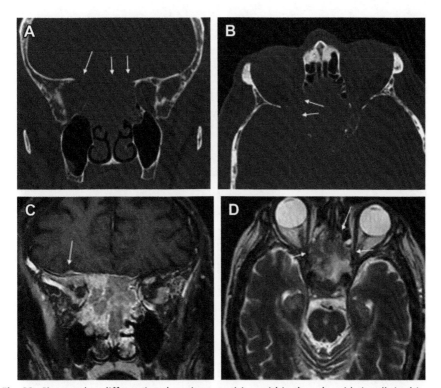

Fig. 22. Sinonasal undifferentiated carcinoma arising within the ethmoid air cells in this patient who presented with headaches and congestion. Coronal (*A*) and axial (*B*) CT images show complete obliteration of the fovea ethmoidalis and cribriform plate, with no distinction on CT between soft-tissue mass and overlying frontal lobes within the anterior cranial fossa (*arrows*). There is also osseous destruction of the right superomedial orbital wall. Coronal fat-suppressed, contrast-enhanced MR image (*C*) demonstrates dural enhancement along the floor of the right anterior cranial fossa (*arrow*). Axial T2-weighted image (*D*) demonstrates amorphous, poorly defined T2-dark signal associated with this highly cellular and infiltrative neoplasm (*arrows*).

and 10% within the ethmoid air cells (**Fig. 21**).[15] Sinonasal undifferentiated carcinoma (SNUC) is a particularly aggressive form of nonsquamous cell carcinoma that most commonly arises within the ethmoid air cells and demonstrates infiltrative, poorly defined margins (**Fig. 22**). Though less common, metastasis or lymphoma can also involve the paranasal sinuses with aggressive, destructive features on imaging. Whereas CT best demonstrates osseous destruction, contrast-enhanced MRI with small-field-of-view fat-saturated pulse sequences optimally demonstrates the extent of intracranial or intraorbital involvement. Highly cellular neoplasms such as sinonasal squamous cell carcinoma, SNUC, and certain metastases will also demonstrate a characteristic T2-dark signal, which can be readily differentiated on MRI from the associated T2-bright secretions retained within the obstructed sinuses (see **Fig. 21**; **Fig. 23**). Subtle enhancement of dura or cranial nerves on MRI suggests intracranial or perineural involvement.

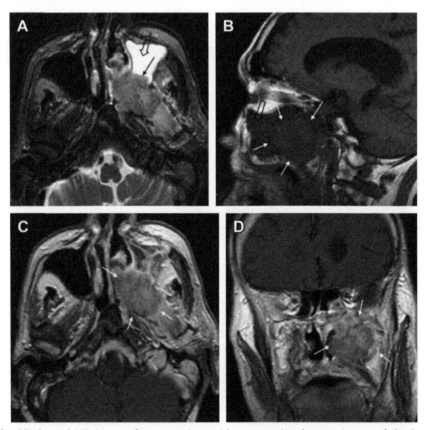

Fig. 23. Several MR images from a patient with metastatic adenocarcinoma of the lung demonstrating a large soft-tissue mass centered within left pterygopalatine fossa extending into posterior left maxillary sinus with destruction of the sinus chamber walls. Cellular soft-tissue mass is dark on T2 (*arrow in A*) and is therefore well distinguished from the adjacent T2-bright, T1-dark retained serous secretions within the obstructed left maxillary sinus (*open arrow in A, B*). Mass demonstrates intermediate signal on precontrast T1-weighted image (*arrows in B*) with enhancement following contrast administration (*arrows in C, D*) suggesting vascularity.

REFERENCES

1. Rosenfeld R, Andes D, Bhattacharyya N, et al. Clinical practice guideline: adult sinusitis. Otolaryngol Head Neck Surg 2007;137(Suppl 3):S1–131.
2. Grossman RI, Yousem DM. Neuroradiology requisites. 2nd edition. Philadelphia: Elsevier; 2003.
3. Wolff H. Headache and other pain. New York: Oxford University Press; 1948.
4. Tosun F, Gerek M, Ozkaptan Y. Nasal surgery for contact point headaches. Headache 2000;40:237–40.
5. Huang H, Lee T, Huang C, et al. Non-sinusitis-related rhinogenous headache: a ten year experience. Am J Otolaryngol 2008;29:326–32.
6. Patel AM, Kennedy DW, Setzen M, et al. "Sinus headache": rhinogenic headache or migraine? An evidence-based guide to diagnosis and treatment. Int Forum Allergy Rhinol 2013;3:221–30.
7. Wittkopf ML, Beddow PA, Russell PT, et al. Revisiting the interpretation of positive sinus CT findings: a radiological and symptom-based review. Otolaryngol Head Neck Surg 2009;140:306–11.
8. Stewart MG, Johnson RF. Chronic sinusitis: symptoms versus CT scan findings. Curr Opin Otolaryngol Head Neck Surg 2004;12:27–9.
9. Bhattacharyya T, Piccirillo J, Wippold FJ. Relationship between patient-based descriptions of sinusitis and paranasal sinus computed tomographic findings. Arch Otolaryngol Head Neck Surg 1997;123:1189–92.
10. Meltzer EO, Hamilos DL, Hadley JA, et al. Rhinosinusitis: establishing definitions for clinical research and patient care. Otolaryngol Head Neck Surg 2004; 131(Suppl):S1–62.
11. Laine F, Smoker W. The osteomeatal unit and endoscopic sinus surgery: anatomy, variations and imaging findings in inflammatory diseases. AJR Am J Roentgenol 1992;159:849–57.
12. Bhattacharyya N. Do maxillary sinus retention cysts reflect obstructive sinus phenomena? Arch Otolaryngol Head Neck Surg 2000;126:1369–71.
13. Bayonne E, Kania R, Tran P, et al. Intracranial complications of rhinosinusitis. A review, typical imaging data and algorithm of management. Rhinology 2009;47: 59–65.
14. McIntosh D, Mahadevan M. Acute orbital complications of sinusitis: the benefits of magnetic resonance imaging. J Laryngol Otol 2008;122:324–6.
15. Loevner LA, Sonners AI. Imaging of neoplasms of the paranasal sinuses. Neuroimaging Clin N Am 2004;14:625–46.

Medical Management of Adult Headache

Frederick G. Freitag, DO, FAHS[a],*, Fallon Schloemer, DO[b]

KEYWORDS

- Analgesics • Nonsteroidal anti-inflammatory drugs • Triptans
- US consortium guideline • Beta blockers • Anti-epileptic drugs • Natural therapies

KEY POINTS

- Simple analgesics may suffice for migraine with little disability, but triptans are essential for many with migraine.
- Chronic migraine is a complication of episodic migraine with numerous other risk factors.
- Medication overuse of acute treatments plays a critical role in many patients.
- Preventive therapies for migraine are not as effective here, but OnabotulinumtoxinA has strong evidence for efficacy.
- Therapies for tension-type headache are focused on prevention, most commonly with older tricyclic antidepressants. Migraine medications are not typically useful for tension-type headache.

INTRODUCTION

In previous articles it is apparent that not all headaches are the same. Therefore, in examining treatment of headache with medical therapies it is necessary to subdivide headache into its component parts and focus on each individually. In this article, we focus on the primary headache disorders, those in which there is no underlying primary causation, save the patient's own natural physiology and genetics. These are migraine, tension-type headache, and cluster headache, as well as chronic migraine, a complication of episodic migraine, and one that can perplex even headache experts. Treatments focus on evidence-based approaches to management insofar as possible with expert opinion where evidence is insufficient to provide guidance.

Disclosures: Advisory Board: Allergan; Consultant: Nupathe, Revance, Transcept, Zogenix; Research: Allergan, Amgen, GlaxoSmithKline; Speakers Bureau: Allergan, Nautilus Neuroscience, Zogenix.
[a] Department of Neurology, Medical College of Wisconsin, 9200 West Wisconsin Avenue, Milwaukee, WI 53226, USA; [b] Department of Neurology, Froedtert Hospital, Medical College of Wisconsin, 9200 West Wisconsin Avenue, Milwaukee, WI 53226, USA
* Corresponding author.
E-mail address: dhcdoc@gmail.com

Abbreviations	
NSAID	Non-steroidal anti-inflammatory agents
DHE	Dihydroergotamine
SUNCT Syndrome	Short-lasting unilateral neuralgiform headache with conjunctival injection and tearing
TTHA	Tension type headache
CM	Chronic Migraine
MO	Medication Overuse
onaBoNTA	OnabotulinumtoxinA
TCA	Tricyclic antidepressants
SSRI	Serotonin specific reuptake inhibitors
PREEMPT	Phase III REsearch Evaluating Migraine Prophylaxis Therapy

EPISODIC MIGRAINE
Acute Treatment

Acute treatments for migraine are designed to relieve the symptom complex of pain, photophobia, phonophobia, and nausea. Ideally, these treatments provide relief within 2 hours, without recurrence and with minimal adverse events. In 2000, the US Headache Consortium produced an evidence-based guideline for acute treatment and report summary.[1] The guideline has not been updated.

Migraine is highly variable within an individual and in the population. Selection of treatments use stratified care based on levels of disability and symptoms, such as nausea or vomiting. Additionally, selecting treatments or route of administration is based on specific attack characteristics to a stepped care approach within and between attacks.[1] Frequency of use is the limiting factor for these agents, as frequent use leads to medication overuse (MO) and chronification of migraine.

Simple analgesics, combination analgesics, and prescription nonsteroidal anti-inflammatory agents (NSAIDs) (**Table 1**) are considered first-line therapy for migraine.[1] Of the NSAIDs, naproxen may have the least risk of cardiovascular concerns.[2] For those patients who fail to respond to these agents consistently, then oral triptans are used. Triptans are used as first-line agents before analgesics for more severely impacted patients. Nonoral administration of triptans or dihydroergotamine (DHE) is preferred for those who do not respond to oral triptans consistently[3] or have early onset of nausea or vomiting.

Newer Acute Treatments

A number of treatments were not available at the time of the 2000 guideline but have evidence similar to those agents in category A of the guidelines for consistent efficacy and tolerability. One involves innovative delivery improving effectiveness, such as diclofenac powder (Cambia).[4] Three other triptans have come on the market: almotriptan, eletriptan, and frovatriptan, and all bear similarity to the 4 reviewed triptans.[5] A novel tablet design combines sumatriptan and naproxen sodium,[6] altering the pharmacokinetics of both drugs for favorable outcomes. An easy to use method is available especially in the patient with nausea, with a recently approved sumatriptan patch (Zelrix).[7] When a nonoral treatment of migraine is needed in which there is early onset of nausea or if the patient does not have a consistent response to oral triptans, then zolmitriptan nasal spray or subcutaneous administration of sumatriptan without a needle (Sumavel DosePro sumatriptan, zogenix pharmaceuticals, emeryville, CA) is available.[8] The NSAID, ketorolac, is used[9] as a parenteral rescue medication.

Table 1
Selected acute treatments for migraine reviewed in US Headache Consortium guideline evidence

Drug	Quality of Evidence[a]	Clinical Uses[b]	Types and Relative Risk of Adverse Events[c]
Simple analgesics/combination analgesics/nonsteroidal anti-inflammatory drugs			
Acetaminophen	B	Nondisabling migraine	Nonspecific/infrequent
Aspirin	A	First line: mild to moderate migraine	Gastrointestinal and bleeding/occasional
Acetaminophen, aspirin, caffeine	A	First line: mild to moderate migraine	Cardiovascular, gastrointestinal, and bleeding/occasional
Diclofenac potassium	B	First line: mild to moderate migraine	Gastrointestinal and bleeding/occasional
Flurbiprofen	B	First line: mild to moderate migraine	Gastrointestinal and bleeding/occasional
Ibuprofen	A	First line: mild to moderate migraine	Gastrointestinal and bleeding/occasional
Naproxen	B	First line: mild to moderate migraine	Gastrointestinal and bleeding/occasional
Naproxen sodium	A	First line: mild to moderate migraine	Gastrointestinal and bleeding/occasional
Ketorolac IM	B	Rescue therapy/severe migraine with contraindications to 5HT agonists	Gastrointestinal and bleeding/infrequent
5HT 1B/1D agonists			
Naratriptan	A	Migraine nonresponding to analgesics/moderate to severe migraine	Nausea, paresthesia, chest discomfort/infrequent when used early in attack
Rizatriptan	A	Migraine nonresponding to analgesics/moderate to severe migraine	Nausea, paresthesia, chest discomfort/infrequent when used early in attack
Sumatriptan	A	Migraine nonresponding to analgesics/moderate to severe migraine	Nausea, paresthesia, chest discomfort/infrequent when used early in attack
Zolmitriptan	A	Migraine nonresponding to analgesics/moderate to severe migraine	Nausea, paresthesia, chest discomfort/infrequent when used early in attack
Sumatriptan nasal spray	A	Migraine nonresponding to analgesics/moderate to severe migraine	Nausea, paresthesia, chest discomfort unpleasant taste/occasional
Sumatriptan SC	A	Moderate to severe migraine/oral nonresponders/early-onset nausea	Nausea, paresthesia, chest discomfort/frequent

(*continued on next page*)

Drug	Quality of Evidence[a]	Clinical Uses[b]	Types and Relative Risk of Adverse Events[c]
Table 1 *(continued)*			
DHE: intravenous/ intramuscular/ subcutaneous	B	Moderate to severe migraine/oral nonresponders/rescue/ headache recurrence/ bridge therapy for CM and MO	Nausea, paresthesia, chest discomfort/frequent
DHE nasal spray	A	Moderate to severe migraine/oral nonresponders/ headache recurrence	Nausea, paresthesia, chest discomfort, nasal congestion/occasional

Abbreviations: CM, chronic migraine; DHE, dihydroergotamine; IM, intramuscular; MO, medication overuse; SC, subcutaneous.

[a] US Headache Consortium Guideline Evidence Classification. Level A: Medications with well-established efficacy. Level B: Medications that are probably effective.

[b] Opinion of authors.

[c] After US Consortium Headache Guideline evidence with author opinion.

Preventive Treatments

Preventive treatment should be considered[10] if migraine attacks occur 4 or 5 days per month with normal functioning or if there are 2 to 3 migraine days per month that have some impairment or disability. The choice of preventive medications (**Table 2**) has been recently reviewed in 2 evidence-based guidelines.[11,12] These include "natural" treatments and prescriptive agents. The treatments of first choice are 3 beta blockers: propranolol, timolol, and metoprolol; 3 antiepileptic agents: valproic acid, divalproex, and topiramate; the triptan: frovatriptan for preventive treatment of menstrual migraine; and the herbal preparation: Petadolex brand of butterbur (Linpharma Inc. Oldsmar, FL), as it is the only formulation that has been subjected to clinical trials. Other agents can be considered based on comorbidities, patient preference, and tolerability. The doses used for all of these agents should be titrated upward to an effective dose over the first month and maintained for 3 months before considering increasing the dose or changing drugs. Titrating the dose minimizes the adverse event burden, common for many patients. Treatment should reduce the migraine burden optimally, then be maintained for a year before attempting to taper the medications, which occurs over several months. Education of the patient in a headache-healthy lifestyle and nonpharmacologic strategies should be encouraged.

CLUSTER HEADACHE

Given the unilateral nature of cluster headache, it is important to consider in the differential diagnosis paroxysmal hemicrania, short-lasting unilateral neuralgiform headache with conjunctival injection and tearing (SUNCT syndrome), primary stabbing headache, and trigeminal neuralgia. The first 3 of these, along with hemicrania continua, share a preventive treatment response to indomethacin, although they are rare conditions even by comparison with cluster headache.

Acute Treatment

Treatment of cluster headache is primarily pharmacologic. There has been some success with behavioral approaches, occipital nerve procedures, and deep brain

Table 2
Selected agents from American Academy guidelines for preventive prescription drugs including nonsteroidal anti-inflammatory drugs, histaminic agents, and nonprescription supplements and vitamins

Drug	Quality of Evidence[a]	Special Clinical Considerations[b]	Types and Relative Risk of Adverse Events[b]
Alpha agonists			
Clonidine	C	Also used for reducing opioid withdrawal	Fatigue, hypotension/ occasional
Guanfacine	C		Fatigue, hypotension/ occasional
ACE inhibitors			
Lisinopril	C	Maybe useful for preservation of renal function in patients with diabetes	Dizziness/infrequent
ACE blocking agents			
Candesartan	C		Dizziness/infrequent
Antidepressants			
Amitriptyline	B	Coexisting depression	Somnolence, anticholinergic, weight gain/frequent
Venlafaxine	B	Coexisting depression, anxiety, perimenopausal	Sexual dysfunction, mood disorders especially teenagers/infrequent
Antiepileptic agents			
Carbamazepine	C	Coexisting seizure disorder, trigeminal neuralgia	Aplastic anemia, dizziness, somnolence, extreme caution in women of childbearing potential/frequent
Divalproex sodium/ valproate	A	Coexisting mood disorder or seizure disorder	Weight gain, hair loss, tremor, extreme caution in women of childbearing potential/ frequent
Topiramate	A	Coexisting seizure disorder	Mood changes, paresthesias, nephrolithiasis, acute glaucoma, weight loss/ frequent
Beta adrenergic blocking agents			
Atenolol	B		Bradycardia, hypotension/occasional
Metoprolol	A		Hypotension/infrequent
Nadolol	B		Hypotension, mood dish orders/occasional
Nebivolol	C		Hypotension/infrequent
Pindolol	C	Raynaud disease	Hypotension/infrequent
Propranolol	A	Acute anxiety disorder	Hypotension, mood disorder/occasional

(continued on next page)

Table 2
(continued)

Drug	Quality of Evidence[a]	Special Clinical Considerations[b]	Types and Relative Risk of Adverse Events[b]
Timolol	A		Hypotension, mood disorder/occasional
5HT1B/1D agonists			
Frovatriptan	A	Menstrual-associated migraine	Nausea, paresthesia, chest discomfort/infrequent
Naratriptan	B	Menstrual-associated migraine	Nausea, paresthesia, chest discomfort/infrequent
Zolmitriptan	B	Menstrual-associated migraine	Nausea, paresthesia, chest discomfort/infrequent
Herbal therapies			
Feverfew	B	MIG-99 only formulation shown effective	Gastrointestinal/ infrequent
Petasites	A	Petadolux only formulation studied. Processing differences between brands may increase risk of adverse events	Gastrointestinal/ infrequent. Other formulations may contain derivatives that are hepatotoxic.
Histaminic agents			
Cyproheptadine	C	Children, cluster headache, category B in pregnancy	Sedation, weight gain/ occasional
Histamine subcutaneous	B	Cluster headache, must be compounded	Flushing, itching/ infrequent
Hormones			
Estrogen (soy isoflavones, dong quai, and black cohosh)/ estradiol	C	Menstrually associated migraine	Alteration of menstrual blood loss/occasional
Minerals and Vitamins			
Co-Q 10	C		Rare
Magnesium	B	Menstrually associated migraine	Gastrointestinal/ occasional based on formulation
Riboflavin	B		Urine discoloration/ frequent
Nonsteroidal anti-inflammatory drugs			
Flurbiprofen	C	Also menstrually associated migraine	Gastrointestinal and bleeding/occasional
Fenoprofen	B	Also menstrually associated migraine	Gastrointestinal and bleeding/occasional
Ibuprofen	B	Also menstrually associated migraine	Gastrointestinal and bleeding/occasional
Ketoprofen	B	Also menstrually associated migraine	Gastrointestinal and bleeding/occasional

(continued on next page)

Table 2
(continued)

Drug	Quality of Evidence[a]	Special Clinical Considerations[b]	Types and Relative Risk of Adverse Events[b]
Mefenamic acid	C	Also menstrually associated migraine	Gastrointestinal and bleeding/occasional
Naproxen	B	Also menstrually associated migraine	Lowest risk of cardiovascular disease complications, gastrointestinal and bleeding/occasional
Naproxen sodium	B	Also menstrually associated migraine	Lowest risk of cardiovascular disease complications, gastrointestinal and bleeding/occasional

Abbreviation: ACE, angiotensin-converting enzyme.
[a] After the Reports of the Quality Standards Subcommittee of the American Academy of Neurology and the American Headache Society. Level A: Medications with well-established efficacy. Level B: Medications that are probably effective. Level C: Medications that are possibly effective.
[b] Opinion of authors.

stimulation. Given its severity and debilitating features, although attention to acute treatment is important, the focus is on preventive treatment. Both the American Academy of Neurology[13] and the European Federation of Neurologic Societies[14] have published evidence-based recommendations.

The current guidelines (**Table 3**) suggest that 100% oxygen at a rate of 6 to 12 L per minute for up to 15 minutes per attack, subcutaneous injection of sumatriptan, and zolmitriptan nasal spray are the first-line treatments for the acute treatment of cluster headache. Oxygen is the treatment of choice, given its side-effect profile and safety; however, the triptans may be more effective acute medications and can be used with greater convenience. Rapid onset of action is essential. This makes injectable and intranasal formulations preferred over the oral triptans. There is limited evidence for the local anesthetic agents lidocaine and cocaine being effective. There is no evidence for the opioid analgesics.

Preventive Treatment

Cluster headache may occur multiple times per day over weeks to months or longer, limiting the use of acute therapies as sole treatment. Preventive therapy (**Table 4**) is a coexisting first-line approach with the acute treatments. The goals of preventive therapy are to decrease the number of attacks and maintain remission over the cluster period. Short courses of corticosteroids are often combined with one of the evidence-based treatments described later in this article, with verapamil being the most common. Once a remission occurs, the steroid is tapered and stopped and the verapamil, for example, is continued at an effective dose until the cluster period has ceased.

Although patients with episodic cluster headache respond readily to treatment, patients with chronic cluster may develop tolerance to treatment requiring other medical treatments, combination treatments, and alternative therapeutic approaches.

Table 3
Acute treatment for cluster headache

Drug/Route of Administration	Quality of Evidence[a]	Comments[b]	Types and Relative Risk of Adverse Events[b]
Oxygen 100% at 6–12 L/min non rebreathing mask	A	Response in 5–15 min, can be repeated as needed, can't easily transport. Despite evidence, not covered by Medicare some other insurance carriers.	Drying effects/rare
Sumatriptan subcutaneous 4–6 mg	A	Limits of 12 mg per day	Nausea, paresthesia, chest discomfort/ frequent
Sumatriptan nasal spray 20 mg	B		Nausea, paresthesia, chest discomfort, taste issues/ frequent
Zolmitriptan nasal spray 5 mg	A	Limits 10–20 mg per day	Nausea, paresthesia, chest discomfort/ frequent
Zolmitriptan oral 5 to 10 mg	A	Limits to 10–20 mg day	Nausea, paresthesia, chest discomfort/ occasional
Lidocaine 4%–10% aqueous/cocaine 10% intranasal	B	Limit to several times per day. Low but defined risk of dependency with cocaine	Paresthesia, altered sense of smell/ frequent

[a] After the American Academy of Neurology and The European Federation of Neurologic Societies guidelines. A = multiple well-controlled trials with consistent response; B = inconsistent response in trials or issues of number and size of trials.
[b] Opinions and recommendations of the authors.

Therapeutic Options in Treatment-Resistant Cluster Headache

When standard pharmacologic treatment fails, there are other therapies that can be considered. Medically these include DHE infusion[15] and histamine desensitization, popularized by Horton and colleagues[16] for cluster headache and shown to be effective for chronic cluster headache.[17] Although out of favor, recent studies[18] of DHE for migraine have been efficacious. There is considerable interest in procedural methods as treatments for intractable cluster headache. These include radiofrequency thermocoagulation,[19] gamma knife radiosurgery,[20] and neuromodulation in the form of deep brain stimulation,[21] occipital nerve stimulation,[22] and sphenopalatine stimulation[23] as treatments.

TREATMENT OF CHRONIC DAILY HEADACHE

Chronic daily headache compromises variant situations from the more common episodic versions of the disorders. There is chronic migraine (CM), chronic cluster, and chronic tension-type headache (TTHA). The treatment of chronic cluster blends with that of episodic and has been discussed. The most common of these is chronic TTHA followed closely by CM. The evolution of symptoms in migraine and tension type with development of chronicity cause these 2 disorders to seem to be more similar than different, the difference being the antecedent headaches before the chronification of the headaches. Patients with frequent headaches are likely to treat their attacks

Table 4
Preventive therapy of cluster headache

Drug	Quality of Evidence[a]	Comments[b]	Types and Relative Risk of Adverse Events[b]
Baclofen 15–30 mg PO	C		Sedation/infrequent
Capsaicin intranasal	C	Civamide an experimental derivative has A-level evidence	Severe burning pain/ frequent
Lithium 600–1500 mg daily	C	Need to monitor renal and thyroid function, especially in treatment of chronic phase. Monitor levels	Hypothyroidism, tremor, cognitive slowing/ frequent
Melatonin 10 mg PO	C		Sedation/frequent
Corticosteroids			
Methylprednisolone 100 mg PO to start and taper	A	Long used on expert opinion with excellent response. Not well tolerated for long-term treatment or sole treatment, headache recurs at physiologic replacement (prednisone 20 mg/d)	Few with short-term use other than increased energy and appetite. Long-term use leads to fluid retention, weight gain, glucose intolerance, cataracts/ frequent. Aseptic necrosis of hip/rare
Prednisone 20 mg/d	Not effective		
Suboccipital steroid injection	B	Usually combined with local anesthetic. This may effective by itself. Must be trained in technique	Pain, neck weakness/ infrequent
Topamax 100 mg/d PO	B	Titrate dose but faster than for migraine.	Mood changes, paresthesias, nephrolithiasis, acute glaucoma, weight loss/ infrequent
Valproic acid 5–20 mg/kg PO daily	C	Conflicting guidance	Weight gain, hair loss, tremor/infrequent
Verapamil 240–960 mg PO	A/C	Conflicting evidence evaluation but is current agent of first choice for episodic and chronic cluster headache clinically	Constipation. Fluid retention. Monitor EKG with doses 480 mg/d or greater.

Abbreviations: EKG, electrocardiogram; PO, by mouth.
[a] After the American Academy of Neurology and The European Federation of Neurologic Societies guidelines. A = multiple well-controlled trials with consistent response; B = inconsistent response in trials or issues of number and size of trials.
[b] Opinions and recommendations of the authors.

of headache as they occur. Unfortunately, the use of acute medications frequently in patients with frequent or CM and TTHA can produce a complication, MO headache.

MO Headache and Acute Treatments

One of the major treatment issues in these chronic disorders is MO and MO headache. In the older literature this is often called rebound headache. MO headache can be defined only by eliminating the overuse of the offending medication(s) and observing an improvement in the patient's headache, which occurs over the coming weeks to several months. This improvement occurs in the absence of other therapeutics being applied to treatment and occurs in approximately 50% of patients[24] with MO. The term rebound headache is a useful description of what a patient experiences when the offending medication causing MO headache is discontinued: the headache pain the patient experiences accelerates for a period of time. MO headache rarely occurs in patients with chronic cluster headache or rare daily headache disorders, such as new daily persistent headache.[24] Overuse of medication must occur for at least 3 consecutive months. MO headache is also defined by the medication taken (**Table 5**). Medication overuse by contrast is the state of affairs in which the patient is taking sufficient acute medications for a long enough period time to develop MO headache, but it is not necessary to "detox" the patient first to determine if MO headache is present before addressing the underlying primary headache disorder.

Other than for a small study[25] of naproxen sodium alone or combined with sumatriptan, there are no trials of acute medications used for migraine and TTHA in patients with chronic headache. That being noted, there is no evidence that the medications used for the acute treatment of each of these disorders has any different efficacy or tolerability in episodic versus chronic form of these headache types. Therefore, other than for limitations to avoid MO, the acute treatment in CM and chronic TTHA are the same agents used for the episodic forms of these disorders.

Preventive Treatment of CM

There are no evidence-based guidelines for the preventive treatment of CM. There are also a limited number of studies that assess preventive treatments for this evolutive state of migraine. Patients do not begin with CM. They have a history of episodic migraine, and over time progress to 15 or more headache days per month. There are risk factors for this. Some of these can be changed and have an impact on development of CM. These include frequent use of acute medications, headache frequency, sleep disorders, psychological issues, and obesity[26] and can impact long-term management of frequent migraine.

There is only one medical therapy that is approved by the Food and Drug Administration (FDA) for the preventive treatment of CM: OnabotulinumtoxinA (OnaBoNTA). It has been subject to clinical trials since 1997.[27] The Phase III REsearch Evaluating Migraine Prophylaxis Therapy (PREEMPT) trials[28,29] were designed for treatment of CM. Previous studies of OnaBoNTA failed to demonstrate evidence for efficacy in other headache disorders, including migraine occurring fewer than 15 days per month.

Table 5
Acute medication allowance to avoid medication overuse

Drug (Dose if Applicable)	Allowed Frequency of Use
Ergotamine (does not include dihydroergotamine), triptans	10 d/mo
Simple analgesics, nonsteroidal anti-inflammatory drugs	15 d/mo
Opioid class analgesics	10 d/mo
Combinations (eg, 2 simple analgesics together, simple analgesic combined with caffeine, triptan combined with nonsteroidal anti-inflammatory drug)	10 d/mo
Caffeine 200 mg/d	None (defined by occurrence of headache within 24 h after discontinuation)

OnaBoNTA injections were given every 12 weeks, the first 2 treatments in the study were placebo controlled and demonstrated significant efficacy over placebo. Patients from the placebo trial enrolled in a long-term study demonstrating continuing efficacy over a year-long treatment. Traditionally, the impression has been that patients with MO will not improve until the MO has been resolved. The PREEMPT study demonstrated that even in patients with MO there was significant improvement across almost all parameters at the 24-week end point.[30]

The FDA-approved protocol for administration of onaBoNTA is the same one used in the PREEMPT trials (**Table 6**). Although the injection procedure is not complex, it does require specific training. This is important for both efficacy and to ensure minimization of adverse events. Examination of other toxin formulations[31] do not make it possible to determine equivalent doses and there is no evidence for other toxin formulations having efficacy.[32] Although OnaBoNTA is the only FDA-approved drug for CM, many insurance companies require patients to have been treated with other drugs with demonstrated efficacy in episodic migraine to receive prior authorization for this therapy. Several agents have been studied in comparator trials to OnaBoNTA.[33–36]

There have been several trials in which combinations of propranolol and topiramate have been studied in different trial designs. Although one study suggested efficacy,[37] the other was terminated for lack of response.[38] Topiramate was studied by itself to determine if it was effective in preventing migraine evolution from a very frequent state of 9 to 14 migraine days per month to CM.[39] Topiramate demonstrated superiority to placebo but did not reach statistical superiority. In those with CM, topiramate demonstrates a modest but statistically significant improvement in outcome parameters[40] both in patients with and without MO headache.[41] A comparator trial of topiramate and divalproex sodium[42] showed both agents providing comparable efficacy and tolerability. Divalproex sodium in an open-label study[43] found 67% of patients on divalproex had at least a 50% reduction in their chronic migraines. A third of patients experienced adverse events. Subsequently, a small double-blind trial demonstrated statistically significant benefit.[44]

Antidepressants in CM and Chronic TTHA

Antidepressants have a long history of use in treating a variety of headache disorders, including CM. In part, this use occurred because of a link between headaches and depression and an idea first propagated by Diamond.[45] The evidence fails to find

---

Table 6
Injection paradigm for use of OnaBoNTA in CM (after PREEMT studies)

OnaBoNTA 200 Units Diluted in 4 mL Preservative-Free Normal Saline Solution. Administer with 31-gauge $^1/_2$-inch Needle

Site	No. Injections	No. Units per Injection
Corrugator muscle	2 (1 each side)	5
Procerus muscle	1	5
Frontalis muscle	4 (2 each side)	5
Temporalis muscle	8 (4 each side)	5
Occipitalis muscle	6 (3 each side)	5
Upper cervical paraspinal muscles	4 (2 each side)	5
Trapezius muscle	6 (3 each side)	5

Abbreviations: CM, chronic migraine; OnaBoNTA, OnabotulinumtoxinA; PREEMPT, Phase III REsearch Evaluating Migraine Prophylaxis Therapy.

a correlation between depressive or other psychiatric symptoms and response to antidepressants.[46]

Optimized treatment of chronic headache[47] showed that a combination of pharmacologic and nonpharmacologic strategies was most likely to produce clinically meaningful improvement. Of the antidepressants used in CM, tricyclic antidepressants (TCAs) are the most commonly used, but few have been subjected to well-designed clinical trials. Results are clouded by definitional terms that have changed over the decades of their use in describing and differentiating CM from TTHA, for example. Amitriptyline has been studied, but the results are mixed and clouded by a high placebo response.[48] To overcome issues of small clinical trials and the wide variety of agents, several meta-analyses have been conducted. One[49] studied 38 trials involving 44 different agents against placebo and demonstrated robust outcomes for all of the antidepressant classes in migraine as well as TTHA. The Cochrane Database[50] report suggested better efficacy for TCA over the serotonin-specific agents without an increased risk of adverse events. Although amitriptyline is the most commonly used, other options exist that can be effective and potentially better tolerated. Positive findings in uncontrolled or small trials have been reported for protriptyline, which is nonsedating and does not cause weight gain,[51] doxepin,[52] and imipramine.[53] Although there are no trials of nortriptyline, it is the active metabolite of amitriptyline and is less sedating and causes less weight gain than amitriptyline. In the elderly, the preference is for doxepin, which has significant effects on central modulation pain without anticholinergic adverse events. A nasal spray formulation demonstrated robust activity in CM in a small unpublished study.[54]

Higher doses of fluoxetine and the serotonin norepinephrine reuptake inhibitor (SNRI) venlafaxine can be alternatives, especially for patients with comorbid depression or perimenopausal symptoms. There is one controlled trial of tizanidine in which it proved equally efficacious in CM as TTHA. Although it is a muscle relaxant, its effects on the trigeminal nucleus caudalis on reducing central spread of pain impulses may account for its benefit.[55] The use of neurostimulation[56] has been applied, as have surgical approaches.[57] These are not advocated in all but exceptional situations at this time.

Treatment of Tension Headache

Patients with infrequent episodic TTHA do not typically present for treatment, as the attacks are self-limited and responsive to over-the-counter remedies and are not discussed further. There are a number of approaches to the treatment of TTHA based on headache frequency and modalities including acute treatments, preventive medical therapies, and nonpharmacologic approaches. The acute medications for TTHA are directed at pain relief. Because the pain of TTHA is typically mild to moderate, the use of opioids is avoided in this headache disorder. All analgesics should be limited to avoid MO. Acetaminophen, aspirin, and the over-the-counter NSAIDs are evidence-based primary options.[58] Use of any single agent should be limited to fewer than 15 days per month to avoid MO. Studies of combination analgesic agents with caffeine have proven effective in clinical trials.[59,60] A meta-analysis[61] of low-strength NSAIDs was comparable to acetaminophen. The use of skeletal muscle relaxants is merely anecdotal, with no controlled trials in TTHA.

In those with frequent headache, preventive medications may be in order. The mainstay of preventive treatment in TTHA is the antidepressant medications.[47] There is a paucity of controlled trials with these agents, and many are intermixed with other chronic daily headaches, such as CM. Practically though, these agents are most likely to improve chronic TTHA. The antidepressants fall into several major groups: TCAs,

| Table 7 | | | |
| Comparator trials of OnaBoNTA in CM | | | |
Comparator Drug	Efficacy	Tolerability	Notes
Topiramate	Similar	OnaBoNTA improved tolerability	2 clinical trials with similar findings
Divalproex	Similar	OnaBoNTA better tolerability.	30% discontinued divalproex vs 3% OnaBoNTA
Amitriptyline	Similar	Similar	250 units OnaBoNTA vs 25–50 mg amitriptyline

Abbreviations: CM, chronic migraine; OnaBoNTA, OnabotulinumtoxinA.

monoamine oxidase inhibitors, and serotonin-specific reuptake inhibitors and the SNRI and other novel antidepressants. The TCA group has the best evidence[58] for clinical efficacy for TTHA. There is supportive evidence[58] for the newer antidepressants venlafaxine and mirtazapine.

The nonpharmacologic technique for TTHA with best evidence for efficacy is the combination of biofeedback along with cognitive behavioral counseling.[62] These techniques focus on not just stress but on muscle relaxation training to reduce pain. Although popular with many patients, there is limited evidence for massage, physical therapy, and manual therapies, such as chiropractic treatment. Acupuncture has a long history of use. An analysis of 120 studies in TTHA suggested that study methods contributed to relative lack of consistent effects.[63] The meta-analysis showed that sham and real acupuncture were equally effective. A group of 43 studies lent themselves to meta-analysis and found electro-acupuncture was more efficacious than manual acupuncture and that needle retention of 30 minutes was more effective than immediate withdrawal. These studies also suggested that twice-a-week treatment was more effective than other schedules. There is no evidence from controlled clinical trials that OnaBoNTA is effective (**Table 7**).[64,65]

SUMMARY

Treatment of headache can appear to be a daunting task. Establishing the diagnosis is the major key, however, to an effective regimen of therapy. Headache frequency and impact provide the next break point. Low frequency, nondisabling headaches can be managed with as-needed over-the-counter remedies. As impact increases, prescriptive specific therapies for the acute attacks becomes necessary based on the original diagnosis. As frequency increases, treatment with top-tier evidence-based preventive therapies enters the picture and stays there even if the headaches are occurring more than 15 days per month, because, save for beta blockers and onaBoNTA, the preventive therapies for the baseline headache disorder are likely to provide at least some benefit at the chronic stage. The vast majority of headaches presenting on self or primary referral in an otorhinolaryngology practice can be managed without additional referral.

REFERENCES

1. Silberstein SD. Practice parameter: evidence-based guidelines for migraine headache (an evidence-based review). Report of the Quality Standards Subcommittee of the American Academy of Neurology. Neurology 2000;55:754–62.

2. Coxib and traditional NSAID Trialists' (CNT) Collaboration, Bhala N, Emberson J, Merhi A, et al. Vascular and upper gastrointestinal effects of non-steroidal anti-inflammatory drugs: meta-analyses of individual participant data from randomised trials. Lancet 2013. http://dx.doi.org/10.1016/S0140-6736(13)60900-9.

3. Diamond S, Freitag FG, Feoktistov A, et al. Sumatriptan 6 mg subcutaneous as an effective migraine treatment in patients with cutaneous allodynia who historically fail to respond to oral triptans. J Headache Pain 2007;8:13–8.

4. Lipton RB, Grosberg B, Singer RP, et al. Efficacy and tolerability of a new powdered formulation of diclofenac potassium for oral solution for the acute treatment of migraine: results from the International Migraine Pain Assessment Clinical Trial (IMPACT). Cephalalgia 2010;30:1336–45.

5. Ferrari MD, Roon KI, Lipton RB, et al. Oral triptans (serotonin 5-HT(1B/1D) agonists) in acute migraine treatment: a meta-analysis of 53 trials. Lancet 2001;358: 1668–75.

6. Khoury CK, Couch JR. Sumatriptan-naproxen fixed combination for acute treatment of migraine: a critical appraisal. Drug Des Devel Ther 2010;4:9–17.

7. Rapoport AM, Freitag F, Pearlman SH. Innovative delivery systems for migraine: the clinical utility of a transdermal patch for the acute treatment of migraine. CNS Drugs 2010;24:929–40.

8. Brandes JL, Cady RK, Freitag FG, et al. Needle-free subcutaneous sumatriptan (Sumavel DosePro): bioequivalence and ease of use. Headache 2009;49: 1435–44.

9. Taggart E, Doran S, Kokotillo A, et al. Ketorolac in the treatment of acute migraine: a systematic review. Headache 2013;53:277–87.

10. Lipton R, Bigal M, Diamond ML, et al. Migraine prevalence, disease burden, and the need for preventive therapy. Neurology 2007;68:343–9.

11. Silberstein SD, Holland S, Freitag F, et al. Evidence-based guideline update: pharmacologic treatment for episodic migraine prevention in adults. Neurology 2012;78:1337–45.

12. Holland S, Silberstein SD, Freitag F, et al. Evidence-based guideline update: NSAIDs and other complementary treatments for episodic migraine prevention in adults. Neurology 2012;78:1346–53.

13. Francis GF, Becker WJ, Pringsheim TM. Acute and preventive pharmacologic treatment of cluster headache. Neurology 2010;75:463–73.

14. May A, Leone M, Afra J, et al. EFNS guidelines on the treatment of cluster headache and other trigeminal-autonomic cephalalgias. Eur J Neurol 2006;13: 1069–73.

15. Mather PJ, Silberstein SD, Schulman EA, et al. The treatment of cluster headache with repetitive intravenous dihydroergotamine. Headache 1991;31: 525–32.

16. Horton BT, Peters GA, Blumenthal LS. A new product in the treatment of migraine: a preliminary report. Proc Staff Meet Mayo Clin 1945;20:241–8.

17. Diamond S, Freitag FG, Diamond ML, et al. Histamine desensitization therapy in intractable cluster headache. Headache Q 1998;9:55–9.

18. Millán-Guerrero RO, Isais-Millán R, Benjamín TH, et al. N-alpha-methyl histamine safety and efficacy in migraine prophylaxis: phase III study. Can J Neurol Sci 2006;33:195–9.

19. Narouze SN. Role of sphenopalatine ganglion neuroablation in the management of cluster headache. Curr Pain Headache Rep 2010;14:160–3.

20. Kano H, Kondziolka D, Niranjan A, et al. γ knife stereotactic radiosurgery in the management of cluster headache. Curr Pain Headache Rep 2011;15:118–23.

21. Fontaine D, Lazorthes Y, Mertens P, et al. Safety and efficacy of deep brain stimulation in refractory cluster headache; a randomized placebo-controlled double-blind trial followed by a 1-year open extension. J Headache Pain 2010;11:23–31.
22. Mueller O, Diener HC, Dammann P, et al. Occipital nerve stimulation for intractable chronic cluster headache or migraine: a critical analysis of direct treatment costs and complications. Cephalalgia 2013. http://dx.doi.org/10.1177/0333102413493193.
23. Tepper SJ, Stillman MJ. Cluster headache: potential options for medically refractory patients (when all else fails). Headache 2013;53:1183–90.
24. Headache Classification Committee of the International Headache Society (IHS). The international classification of headache disorders, 3rd edition (beta version). Cephalalgia 2013;33:629–808.
25. Dexter JK, Cady RK, Nett R, et al. Treatment of chronic migraine: a three-month comparator study of naproxen sodium vs. SumaRT/Nap. Cephalalgia 2013; 33(Suppl 8):53–4.
26. Silberstein SD, Dodick D, Freitag F, et al. Pharmacological approaches to managing migraine and associated comorbidities—clinical considerations for monotherapy versus polytherapy. Headache 2007;47:585–99.
27. Hobson DE, Gladish DF. Botulinum toxin injection for cervicogenic headache. Headache 1997;37:253–5.
28. Diener HC, Dodick DW, Aurora SK, et al. OnabotulinumtoxinA for treatment of chronic migraine: results from the double-blind, randomized, placebo-controlled phase of the PREEMPT 2 trial. Cephalalgia 2010;30:804–14.
29. Aurora SK, Dodick DW, Turkel CC, et al. OnabotulinumtoxinA for treatment of chronic migraine: results from the double-blind, randomized, placebo-controlled phase of the PREEMPT 1 trial. Cephalalgia 2010;30:793–803.
30. Silberstein SD, Blumenfeld AM, Cady RK, et al. OnabotulinumtoxinA for treatment of chronic migraine: PREEMPT 24-week pooled subgroup analysis of patients who had acute headache medication overuse at baseline. J Neurol Sci 2013;331:48–56.
31. Schulte-Mattler WJ, Martinez-Castrillo JC. Botulinum toxin therapy of migraine and tension-type headache: comparing different botulinum toxin preparations. Eur J Neurol 2006;13(Suppl 1):51–4.
32. Schulte-Mattler WJ, Krack P. Treatment of chronic tension-type headache with botulinum toxin A: a randomized, double-blind, placebo-controlled multicenter study. Pain 2004;109:110–4.
33. Mathew NT, Jaffri SF. Double-blind comparison of OnabotulinumtoxinA (BOTOX) and topiramate (TOPAMAX) for the prophylactic treatment of chronic migraine: a pilot study. Headache 2009;49:1466–78.
34. Cady RK, Schreiber CP, Porter JA, et al. A multi-center double-blind pilot comparison of OnabotulinumtoxinA and topiramate for the prophylactic treatment of chronic migraine. Headache 2011;51:21–32.
35. Blumenfeld AM, Schim JD, Chippendale TJ. Botulinum toxin type A and divalproex sodium for prophylactic treatment of episodic or chronic migraine. Headache 2008;48:210–20.
36. Magalhães E, Menezes C, Cardeal M, et al. Botulinum toxin type A versus amitriptyline for the treatment of chronic daily migraine. Clin Neurol Neurosurg 2010;112:463–6.
37. Pascual J, Rivas MT, Leira R. Testing the combination beta-blocker plus topiramate in refractory migraine. Acta Neurol Scand 2007;115:81–3.

38. Silberstein SD, Dodick DW, Lindblad AS, et al. Randomized, placebo-controlled trial of propranolol added to topiramate in chronic migraine. Neurology 2012;78: 976–84.
39. Lipton RB, Silberstein S, Dodick D, et al. Topiramate intervention to prevent transformation of episodic migraine: the topiramate INTREPID study. Cephalalgia 2011;31:18–30.
40. Diener HC, Bussone G, Van Oene JC, et al. Topiramate reduces headache days in chronic migraine: a randomized, double-blind, placebo-controlled study. Cephalalgia 2007;27:814–23.
41. Silberstein S, Lipton R, Dodick D, et al. Topiramate treatment of chronic migraine: a randomized, placebo-controlled trial of quality of life and other efficacy measures. Headache 2009;49:1153–62.
42. Bartolini M, Silvestrini M, Taffi R, et al. Efficacy of topiramate and valproate in chronic migraine. Clin Neuropharmacol 2005;28:277–9.
43. Freitag FG, Diamond S, Diamond ML, et al. Divalproex in the long-term treatment of chronic daily headache. Headache 2001;41:271–8.
44. Yurekli VA, Akhan G, Kutluhan S, et al. The effect of sodium valproate on chronic daily headache and its subgroups. J Headache Pain 2008;9:37–41.
45. Diamond S. Depressive headaches. Headache 1964;4:255–60.
46. Smitherman TA, Walters AB, Maizels M, et al. The use of antidepressants for headache prophylaxis. CNS Neurosci Ther 2011;17:462–9.
47. Holroyd KA, O'Donnell FJ, Stensland M, et al. Management of chronic tension-type headache with tricyclic antidepressant medication, stress management therapy, and their combination: a randomized controlled trial. JAMA 2001;285: 2208–15.
48. Couch JR. Amitriptyline in the prophylactic treatment of migraine and chronic daily headache. Headache 2011;51:33–51.
49. Tomkins GE, Jackson JL, O'Malley PG, et al. Treatment of chronic headache with antidepressants: a meta-analysis. Am J Med 2001;111:54–63.
50. Moja PL, Cusi C, Sterzi RR, et al. Selective serotonin re-uptake inhibitors (SSRIs) for preventing migraine and tension-type headaches. Cochrane Database Syst Rev 2005;(3):CD002919.
51. Cohen GL. Protriptyline, chronic tension-type headaches, and weight loss in women. Headache 1997;37:433–6.
52. Morland TJ, Storli OV, Mogstad TE. Doxepin in the prophylactic treatment of mixed "vascular" and tension headache. Headache 1979;19:382–3.
53. Elser JM, Woody RC. Migraine headache in the infant and young-child. Headache 1990;30:366–8.
54. Winston Pharmaceuticals. Doxepin. Available at: http://www.winstonlabs.com/productdevelopment/doxepin.asp. Accessed July 14, 2013.
55. Saper JR, Lake AE 3rd, Cantrell DT, et al. Chronic daily headache prophylaxis with tizanidine: a double-blind, placebo-controlled, multicenter outcome study. Headache 2002;42:470–82.
56. Reed KL. Peripheral neuromodulation and headaches: history, clinical approach, and considerations on underlying mechanisms. Curr Pain Headache Rep 2013;17:305–14.
57. Guyuron B, Kriegler JS, Davis J, et al. Five-year outcome of surgical treatment of migraine headaches. Plast Reconstr Surg 2011;127:603–8.
58. Bendtsen L, Evers S, Linde M, et al. EFNS guideline on the treatment of tension-type headache—report of an EFNS task force. Eur J Neurol 2010; 17:1318–25.

59. Rabello GD, Forte LV, Galvao AC. Clinical evaluation of the efficacy of the para-cetamol and caffeine combination in the treatment of tension headache. Arq Neuropsiquiatr 2000;58:90–8.
60. Diamond S, Balm TK, Freitag FG. Ibuprofen plus caffeine in the treatment of tension-type headache. Clin Pharmacol Ther 2000;68:312–9.
61. Yoon YJ, Kim JH, Kim SY, et al. A comparison of efficacy and safety of non-steroidal anti-inflammatory drugs versus acetaminophen in the treatment of episodic tension-type headache: a meta-analysis of randomized placebo-controlled trial studies. Korean J Fam Med 2012;33:262–71.
62. Andrasik F. Behavioral treatment approaches to chronic headache. Neurol Sci 2003;24(Suppl 2):S80–5.
63. Hao XA, Xue CC, Dong L, et al. Factors associated with conflicting findings on acupuncture for tension-type headache: qualitative and quantitative analyses. J Altern Complement Med 2013;19:285–97.
64. Freitag FG. Preventative treatment for migraine and tension-type headaches: do drugs having effects on muscle spasm and tone have a role? CNS Drugs 2003; 17:373–81.
65. Gobel H, Heinze A, Heinze-Kuhn K, et al. Evidenced based medicine: botulinum toxin A in migraine and tension type headache. J Neurol 2001;248(Suppl 1): 34–8.

What the Nonneurologist Can Do to Treat Headache

Dara G. Jamieson, MD

KEYWORDS

- Migraine headaches • Triptans • Imaging • Treatment
- Trigeminal autonomic cephalalgias

KEY POINTS

- Patients with common primary headache types can be treated by multiple different specialists, including otolaryngologists.
- Most patients with chronic headaches who present for medical evaluation and treatment will have migraine headaches, which afflict approximately 36 million Americans.
- Brain imaging, which is not necessary for most patients with primary headaches, may show unrelated incidental findings.
- Migraines can be treated with lifestyle modification, triptans for acute treatment of pain, and preventive medications to decrease the frequency and severity of headaches.
- Multiple types of side-locked headaches, including those with ipsilateral autonomic symptoms, can be prevented by indomethacin.

OVERVIEW

Headache is a virtually universal experience, with almost everyone experiencing headaches at some time. As a very common complaint causing patients to seek medical consultation, physicians of almost every specialty will hear about headaches from patients, friends, or family. Many of the millions of chronic headache sufferers can and should be treated by nonneurologists, including otolaryngologists. Primary care practitioners, including internists and gynecologists, treat most patients with episodic or uncomplicated headaches. Patients often consult otolaryngologists before any other specialty because they interpret their head or facial pain of migraine as a symptom of sinus or ear disease. Otolaryngologists should be aware of the different common headache types of their patients, as they can often diagnose and initiate treatment.[1] Ophthalmologists are also often consulted initially, when chronic headaches are interpreted as being due to eye strain. Patients may consult with dentists because they interpret headaches or facial pain as being caused by temporomandibular joint pain or tooth disorders.[2,3] The primary headache types of migraine headache, cluster

Clinical Neurology, Weill Cornell Medical College, New York Presbyterian Hospital, 428 East 72nd Street, Suite 400, New York, NY 10021
E-mail address: dgj2001@med.cornell.edu

Otolaryngol Clin N Am 47 (2014) 239–254
http://dx.doi.org/10.1016/j.otc.2013.10.005
0030-6665/14/$ – see front matter © 2014 Elsevier Inc. All rights reserved.

headache, paroxysmal hemicrania, and hemicrania continua may present to dentists with the chief complaint of tooth pain.[4]

PRIMARY AND SECONDARY HEADACHE TYPES

The International Headache Society (ISH) has published systematic definitions of different types of headaches in an effort to improve the diagnosis and treatment of headaches.[5] Headaches are divided broadly into primary and secondary, depending on their cause. Primary headaches, the most common type, are not associated with anatomic or physiologic abnormalities. Most patients who present for medical evaluation will have a type of primary headache, usually migraine headaches. The major primary headaches are migraine (with or without aura), tension-type headache, and trigeminal autonomic cephalgias (TACs). Other more unusual types of primary headache may occur less frequently, especially in individuals prone to headaches of multiple types. Health care providers other than neurologists, including otolaryngologists, can diagnose and treat many patients with primary headache types.

Secondary headaches are due to a distinct and known anatomic, physiologic, inflammatory, vascular or infectious cause. Although they are much less common than primary headaches, secondary headaches should be considered in all patients who present for evaluation of headaches. Patients who have a primary headache disorder may also develop unrelated secondary headaches, so primary headache patients should be questioned about a change in character or frequency of headache that may indicate another superimposed headache type. There are many types of secondary headaches, most of which should be treated in consultation with a neurologist. The underlying disease causing the headaches may require urgent diagnosis and treatment because of the potential complications that can expand beyond head pain. Even if the underlying disease causing secondary headaches does not itself mandate immediate intervention, secondary headaches generally will not resolve until their specific cause is diagnosed and treated. **Box 1** lists some, but not all, red flags indicating that patients should be rapidly triaged to a neurologist for evaluation.

Box 1
Some red flags that indicate need for a neurologic consultation

- Abnormal neurologic examination, including papilledema
- Focal neurologic symptoms that last longer than 30 minutes or do not disappear after headache is over
- A severe headache that is of peak intensity at the very onset of pain
- Unexplainable worsening of previously existing headaches
- Change in character of the patient's typical chronic headaches
- Side-locked headaches that are never bilateral or contralateral
- Headaches that are clearly positional (eg, worse when recumbent), or severely worse with coughing, sneezing, or Valsalva
- New-onset headaches at an older age (>50 years)
- New-onset headaches in patients with active cancer or human immunodeficiency virus infection
- Headache associated with systemic illness (eg, fever, rash, stiff neck)
- Chronic headaches, transient visual changes, pulsatile tinnitus in an obese woman

Causes of secondary headache include mass lesions, such as tumors and vascular lesions, which are generally accompanied by focal neurologic signs and symptoms. Infections, including meningitis, encephalitis, and brain abscess, may present with headache, fever, alteration in consciousness, and focal neurologic signs and symptoms pointing toward the diagnosis of a secondary headache. Headaches with persistent focal neurologic complaints and/or abnormalities on neurologic examination should be referred to a neurologist for further evaluation.

BRAIN IMAGING IN HEADACHE DISORDERS

The issue of appropriate brain imaging in headache patients is problematic, as not all patients with headaches should be imaged. If more than half of all Americans have a headache each year and headache disorders in the United States already result in more than $31 billion in annual direct and indirect economic costs,[6] imaging the entire population with headaches, even once in their lifetime, would be impractical and an exorbitant waste of resources. Estimating which patients are likely to have a clinically relevant brain lesion causing headaches is crucial to avoid both unnecessary imaging and unnecessary detection of incidental and clinically irrelevant lesions. In patients without focal neurologic abnormalities on examination who appear to have a primary headache, the yield of brain imaging for significant or correlating intracranial findings is generally low. Most patients who present with a history of chronic headaches do not need brain imaging. If the history and physical examination are consistent with migraine or tension-type headache (TTH), and if there are no red flags indicating a possible secondary headache, an imaging procedure is not needed. However, if the patient with a migraine or TTH does not respond as expected to the appropriate treatment, imaging, generally a magnetic resonance imaging (MRI) scan of the brain without contrast, is appropriate.

Indiscriminate imaging often reveals findings without clinical significance that increase anxiety. The incidence of incidental, yet not clinically relevant, brain and head and neck imaging findings in a young healthy population, such as those with primary headaches, is high. An analysis of the MR images obtained from 203 healthy young adult volunteers (mean age 21.9 years; range 18–35 years) found a high prevalence of incidental brain and head and neck abnormalities (9.4% and 36.7%, respectively).[7] All incidental brain findings were clinically silent, not requiring follow-up, and included cysts (pineal gland, arachnoid, Rathke cleft), widened bifrontal subarachnoid space, white matter lesions, and Chiari I malformations. The high occurrence of abnormal findings (36.7%) in the upper head and neck region was mainly explained by simple sinus disease which, when excluded, reduced the incidence to 14.4%. The most common incidental head and neck findings were hyoplastic frontal or maxillary sinuses, sinonasal retention cysts or polyps, mucosal swelling, lymphadenopathy, cystic lesions in the parotid gland, and bilateral osteomeatal abnormality. In older adults, incidental findings on brain MRI are likely to include increased white matter hyperintensities attributable to ischemic small-vessel disease, silent brain infarcts, and incidental neoplasms such as meningiomas.[8] The detection of incidental findings of MRI increases with high resolution sequences in comparison with standard resolution.

Migraine is associated with a significantly increased risk of brain lesions found on MRI, including subclinical infarcts in the posterior circulation, white matter lesions, and brainstem hyperintense lesions.[9] The number of migraine attacks, frequency of migraines, migraine severity, type of migraine headaches, and migraine therapy are not associated with lesion progression. Increase in deep white matter hyperintensity volume on MRI in migraine patients was not significantly associated with worsening cognition.[10] The patient with chronic headaches who is found to have white matter lesions on MRI should be advised that these lesions are unlikely to be of clinical significance. However, referral to a neurologist for consultation may be indicated, in order to discuss the MRI findings and to evaluate for the rare overlap between migraines and other neurologic diseases that can cause white matter lesions in the brain.

Although the likelihood of finding a causal lesion in a suspected primary headache disorder is very small, imaging may be indicated in some patients with primary headache to rule out primary-headache mimics. Criteria that may be used to justify imaging in suspected migraine patients include: unilateral headaches that are always on the same side; headaches associated with aura lasting longer than an hour or an aura that persists after the headache has resolved; and motor or dysphasic auras. In most cases for patients with a suspected migraine or TTH, if a brain imaging study is considered appropriate, an MRI scan of the brain without contrast should be ordered to rule out a causal lesion. When there is a suspicion of a secondary headache, brain imaging with an MRI scan of the brain (or a computed tomography [CT] scan of the head if an MRI is contraindicated) should be obtained, often with contrast enhancement.[11] Patients with most secondary headaches should be treated in consultation with a neurologist.

*A 30-year-old man consulted an otolaryngologist for right frontal throbbing head pain and nasal congestion. The pain, which was never on the left or bilateral, was improved by rest in a quiet, dark room and acetaminophen/aspirin/caffeine combination medication. He had photophobia and phonophobia, but no nausea. He had a chronic cough. He denied ringing in the ears, dizziness, or hearing loss. Nasopharyngeal endoscopy revealed a septum severely deviated to the left, with a large spur with nasal obstruction and inferior turbinate hypertrophy. The neurologic examination was normal. A CT scan of the head and sinuses was interpreted as being normal (**Fig. 1**A–D). Migraine was diagnosed and the patient was treated with a triptan. The throbbing headaches with sensitivity to light and sound increased in frequency. A more detailed history revealed that the patient had bilateral dull headaches behind his eyes without nausea or photophobia/phonophobia, starting as a young boy. Then for about 3 to 4 years he had different headaches with right facial pain lasting up to 2 minutes. About 2 years after his initial evaluation, a neurologist found a left visual field deficit and pupillary asymmetry, with a possible skew deviation and papilledema. An MRI scan showed a large sellar/ suprasellar mass pressing on the chiasm (see **Fig. 1**E, F). A right supraorbital craniotomy for lesional biopsy diagnosed a prolactin-secreting pituitary adenoma.*

MIGRAINE

Most patients who present to a physician for evaluation and treatment of chronic headaches will have migraine headaches. Although headaches span the human life cycle, with infants and centenarians both suffering the effects of migraines, the peak age for migraines is 25 to 55 years. The prevalence of migraine in adults is 18.5%, migraine with aura 4.4%, and chronic migraine 0.5%. The rate of migraine in children is 10.1%, and migraine with aura 1.6%.[12] Most patients who seek medical attention from nonneurologists for chronic headaches producing functional disability have migraine headaches. Migraine headaches are severely disabling, with a distinct pathophysiologic mechanism. While the IHS criteria for the diagnosis of migraine headache (**Box 2**) are useful for research studies on migraine,[5] they are too stringent to encompass all headaches in migraine sufferers. Migraine headaches can be unilateral or bilateral, with pain that can be throbbing or constant. Accompanying gastrointestinal

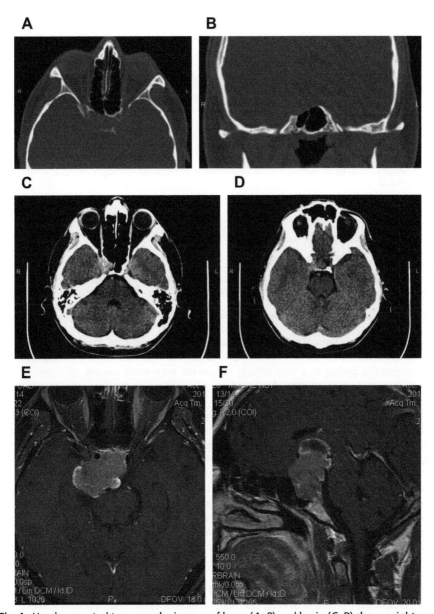

Fig. 1. Head computed tomography images of bone (*A, B*) and brain (*C, D*) show a right parasellar lesion in the region of the cavernous sinus, causing sellar erosion. T1-weighted magnetic resonance images (*E, F*) show a contrast-enhancing mass in the sellar/parasellar region, encasing the right internal carotid artery and compressing the optic chiasm.

symptoms and sensitivities can occur with some, but not all, migraine headaches. Migraine headaches may be triggered in susceptible individuals by environmental stimuli that are innocuous to those who do not suffer migraines. The most common migraine triggers are change in sleep habits (too much or too little sleep), stress or relief from stress, alcohol, change in weather, and hunger and/or dehydration. Some foods may

---

Box 2
International Classification of Headache Disorders (ICHD-3) criteria for migraine without aura

A. At least 5 attacks fulfilling criteria B–D

B. Headache attacks lasting 4 to 72 hours (untreated or unsuccessfully treated)

C. Headache has at least 2 of the following 4 characteristics:

   1. Unilateral location

   2. Pulsating quality

   3. Moderate or severe pain intensity

   4. Aggravation by or causing avoidance of routine physical activity (eg, walking or climbing stairs)

D. During headache at least 1 of the following:

   1. Nausea and/or vomiting

   2. Photophobia and phonophobia

E. Not better accounted for by another ICHD-3 diagnosis

From Headache Classification Committee of the International Headache Society (IHS). The international classification of headache disorders, 3rd edition (beta version). Cephalalgia 2013;33:629–808; with permission.

---

trigger some headaches in some people at some time; in general, however, strict food avoidance has little effect on migraine prevention for most patients. In many women their menstrual period is a very strong trigger for their most severe migraine headaches.[13] Identification of individual triggers by a patient is the first step in migraine prevention.

Most migraines are not accompanied by any focal neurologic symptoms, but some migraine sufferers may have some headaches with a neurologic aura. Migraines with aura are migraine headaches with focal neurologic symptoms (binocular visual disturbances, unilateral numbness, unilateral weakness, speech difficulty) that occur before or during the head pain. The aura generally lasts less than 60 minutes. There may be a symptom-free period of up to 60 minutes before the headache pain begins. The most common aura is binocular alteration in vision, with a scintillating scotoma in the unilateral peripheral vision that increases in size over time (ie, gradual onset) and then suddenly disappears (ie, sudden offset). Specialists other than neurologists are often consulted by patients with migraine, with ophthalmologists seeing patients in whom the new-onset visual aura is more distressing than the accompanying headache.

Vertigo is very common in migraneurs, both in association with headache and occurring in isolation. A temporal overlap between vestibular symptoms, such as vertigo and head-movement intolerance, and migraine symptoms, such as headache, photophobia, and phonophobia, may indicate the diagnosis of vestibular migraine.[14] The symptoms of imbalance and vertigo may overshadow the head pain, leading to initial consultation with an otolaryngologist. Vestibular migraine, recurrent attacks of vertigo caused by migraine, presents with attacks of spontaneous or positional vertigo lasting seconds to days, accompanied by migrainous symptoms. When headache is absent during acute attacks, other migrainous features are identified by history in a patient with a predilection for headaches. By contrast, vestibular testing serves mainly for the exclusion of other diagnoses. Once underlying otologic disease is ruled out, treatment is targeted at the underlying migraine.[15] Caffeine cessation, nortriptyline, and topiramate, treatments used successfully for chronic migraine both with and without aura, have been shown to be effective treatments for migraine-related vertigo.[16]

Patients with frequent or prolonged migraine with aura should generally have a consultation with a neurologist, as patients with migraine with aura have an increased risk of stroke and cardiovascular disease. These patients should be screened for vascular risk factors to determine their individual risk. An increased risk for ischemic stroke has been found in patients with migraine, with the greatest and most consistent increase found in younger women who have migraine with aura. Relative estimates of increased risk range from 3.8 to 8.4. However, the absolute risk of ischemic stroke is small; the estimated attributable risk ranges from 18 to 40 additional cases of ischemic stroke per 100,000 women per year.[17] Oral contraceptives and smoking increase the risk for ischemic stroke in women with migraine with aura. An increased prevalence of patent foramen ovale in patients with migraine with aura has an unclear significance in the pathogenesis of migraine-associated stroke.[18]

Migraine Treatment

Lifestyle modification

Patients have often lived with chronic headaches for years, thinking that having headaches is a normal part of life for which there is no treatment. Recognition of the disability of patients' chronic headaches along with a compassionate, consistent approach to their care can markedly improve the quality of their lives.

The general principles of headache treatment are:

- Establish an accurate diagnosis
- Educate patients about their condition, its treatment, and its natural history
- Establish realistic expectations about headache treatment
- Encourage patients to participate in their own management
  - Adjust lifestyle to avoid headaches
  - Discuss treatment/medication preferences
  - Cooperate with medical treatment recommendations
  - Keep a headache diary to monitor the frequency and severity of headaches

The first step in decreasing the frequency and severity of headaches is a regulated lifestyle with avoidance of headache triggers. Recommended lifestyle modification includes all of the following: regular meals minimizing alcohol and processed foods; the same number of hours of refreshing sleep every night; adequate hydration with water; regular, pleasurable exercise; and avoidance of stress. Any physician consulted by a patient who appears to have migraine headaches can counsel patients on lifestyle modification. **Box 3** lists lifestyle suggestions that can be offered to patients as an initial nonpharmacologic approach to the management of migraine headaches. For many patients, lifestyle management in combination with an effective acute pain medication significantly decreases the disability associated with chronic migraines.

Acute pain medication

Migraine-specific medication to treat acute migraine pain significantly decreases the disability associated with migraines. Many patients treat migraine headaches initially with over-the-counter medications such as nonsteroidal anti-inflammatory drugs (NSAIDs) and combination analgesics such as aspirin/acetaminophen/caffeine. Patients often seek medical help when they become eventually frustrated by the lack of efficacy of these easily obtainable medications, and justifiably concerned about the use excess use of acute pain medications. Medication-overuse headaches can occur with frequent and prolonged use of acute pain medication.

Box 3
Lifestyle modification to decrease headaches

Decrease headaches by:

Avoiding known triggers (ie, stress, foods, alcohol, smells, change in habits) that bring on your headaches

Getting at least 30 minutes of aerobic exercise at least 3 to 4 times weekly

Keeping regular sleeping habits with the same amount of sleep every night of the week

Eating regular meals and drinking water to avoid hunger or dehydration

Decreasing unnecessary stress and being aware that headaches may occur after the stress is over

Trying relaxation techniques, biofeedback, yoga, meditation to decrease the effects of stress

Not smoking; smoking increases the risk of multiple health problems including chronic headaches

Tapering off caffeine-containing drinks (ie, coffee, tea, soda)

Maintaining an ideal body weight through decreased food portions and increased exercise

Decreasing the excessive use of acute pain medication to avoid medication-overuse headaches

---

The most migraine-specific and consistently effective treatment for acute migraine pain is a group of medications called triptans. These serotonin ($5\text{-HT}_{1B/1D}$) receptor agonists are listed in **Box 4**. A triptan for treatment of acute headache pain should be considered for most patients with migraine with and without aura, including children and older adults. The nonneurologist can appropriately prescribe these medications for a patient with episodic migraine, without or with aura, who does not have uncontrolled vascular risk factors or a known history of cardiovascular or cerebrovascular disease. Theoretically these medications should be avoided in migraine patients

---

Box 4
Triptans: serotonin ($5\text{-HT}_{1B/1D}$) receptor agonists

Sumatriptan[a] (Imitrex): oral 25, 50, 100 mg; nasal 5, 20 mg; autoinjector 6 mg, 4 mg

Sumatriptan (Alsuma): autoinjector 6 mg

Sumatriptan (Sumavel DosePro): needle-free delivery system 6 mg

Sumatriptan (Zecuity): iontophoretic transdermal system 6.5 mg/4 hours

Sumatriptan 80 mg/naproxen 550 mg (Treximet): oral

Zolmitriptan[a] (Zomig): oral 2.5, 5 mg; ODT 2.5, 5 mg; nasal 5 mg

Naratritpan[a] (Amerge): oral 1, 2.5 mg

Rizatriptan[a] (Maxalt): oral 5, 10 mg; ODT 5, 10 mg

Almotriptan (Axert): oral 6.25, 12.5 mg

Frovatriptan (Frova): oral 2.5 mg

Eletriptan (Relpax): oral 40 mg

Abbreviation: ODT, orally dissolvable tablet.
[a] Available as a generic medication.

who have auras that last longer than 1 hour or involve focal neurologic complaints other than visual loss or sensory changes. The effective use of triptans includes treating with the medication early in the pain ("like a fire-extinguisher") and using a dose that is high enough to decrease the risk of migraine recurrence. Lower doses of the listed triptans can be used in children, but adolescents and adults should be treated with the higher dose. For patients with severe nausea and vomiting, an orally dissolving tablet or an intranasal or subcutaneous injection may be used. Triptans are generally very well tolerated with very few side effects. Chest discomfort is more common with sumatriptan than with the newer triptans. Lack of response to one triptan does not predict response to another triptan; therefore, multiple triptans may need to be tried before one is found that is effective for each individual migraine patient.[19]

The response to triptan therapy may indicate the diagnosis of patients with migraine headaches who present to otolaryngologists believing they have sinus headache. In a prospective clinical trial using triptans for empiric treatment of sinus headache in patients with endoscopy-negative and CT-negative sinus examinations, 31 of 54 patients (82%) had significant reduction of headache pain with triptan use.[20] Thirty-five patients (92%) who believed they had sinus headaches experienced a significant reduction in headache pain in response to migraine-directed therapy. Seventeen patients (31%) withdrew or failed to follow up, often reluctant to accept a diagnosis of migraine. Clinicians who care for patients with headaches note a frequent reluctance to relinquish the diagnosis of sinus headache when patients are diagnosed with migraine headaches.

Medications containing opioids or butalbital should not be used for the treatment of acute migraine pain, other than under exceptional circumstances.[21] No randomized controlled study of migraine treatment has shown pain-free results with opioids, and multiple adverse physiologic and anatomic effects are associated with opioid exposure. Opioids are pronociceptive, prevent reversal of migraine central sensitization, and interfere with the effectiveness of migraine-specific medications.[22] These types of medications, more so than over-the-counter or other prescription medications used for the treatment of acute pain, increase the risk of medication-overuse headache with escalating frequency of use.[23] Chronic daily headache resulting from medication overuse cannot be treated until the offending agent is withdrawn, usually with the help of a daily preventive medication.[24] Transformation of primary headache types to chronic daily headache because of medication overuse can be prevented by discouraging frequent weekly use of acute pain medication and by encouraging the use of a preventive medication to decrease the frequency and severity of multiple weekly headaches. All physicians who care for patients with chronic headaches should question patients about the specific amounts of acute pain medication consumed per month, and should limit access to medications with habituation potential.

Preventive medications
Patients with episodic migraine who take an acute pain medication a few times a month to control pain are appropriately treated by a nonneurologist. However, when an acute pain medication is needed more than about once a week then a preventive medication, taken every day to decrease the frequency and severity of headaches, may be appropriate for patients in whom migraine headaches are decreasing their quality of life. A migraine sufferer with headaches lasting longer than 4 hours, occurring at least 15 days of the month for three months, is diagnosed with chronic migraines and is appropriate for preventive therapy. For migraine sufferers with frequent headaches, a daily medication can decrease the incidence of headaches, the use of acute medications, and the disability of headaches. Patients often report

improved response to triptans when they are also taking a preventive medication. Medications used to treat seizures, elevated blood pressure, and mood disorders are also used to prevent migraines, as listed in **Box 5**.

The Quality Standards Subcommittee of the American Academy of Neurology and the American Headache Society determined from a literature review that divalproex sodium, sodium valproate, topiramate, metoprolol, propranolol, and timolol are effective for migraine prevention.[25] The choice of preventive medication often depends on how potential side effects would affect the patient's comorbid conditions or symptoms. For example, topiramate may be appropriate for an overweight migraine sufferer, but should be used with caution in patients who are very thin or have a history of renal stones. Propranolol is appropriate for a migraine sufferer with anxiety or elevated blood pressure, but low blood pressure, asthma, diabetes, and depression may be contraindications to the use of a β-blocker. Nortriptyline is effective for the prevention of migraine and TTH and may treat insomnia; however, patients may experience increased appetite and constipation. Although preventive medications are rarely used in pregnant migraine sufferers, valproic acid and divalproex sodium are contraindicated and should not be taken by pregnant women for the prevention of migraine headaches.[26] A triptan with a long half-life, frovatriptan, is effective for prevention of menstrual migraine.[25] Frovatriptan can be taken once or twice a day for about 3 days before the expected menstrual migraine, then continued daily for a total of 6 days until the time of expected headache and menstrual flow. *Petasites hybridus* (butterbur) may be an effective complementary therapy for episodic migraine prevention.[27] OnabotulinumtoxinA toxin can be injected by a headache specialist into muscles in the head, neck, and shoulders of patients with chronic migraines whose headaches are not controlled by oral preventive medications. Patients with frequent migraines who do not respond easily to preventive treatment should be evaluated by a neurologist to determine whether more complicated strategies can decrease their disability caused by migraines.

TENSION-TYPE HEADACHE

TTH is the most common type of primary headache, with lifetime prevalence in the general population of 30% to 78%.[5] There may be a neurobiological basis for the more severe subtypes of TTH, but the exact mechanism is not known. TTH may be episodic or chronic. Most patients treat TTH with over-the-counter medications such as NSAIDs or acetaminophen and do not seek medical attention, but the disability from these headaches can be severe, especially when they evolve from occasional episodic headaches to frequent chronic headaches.

Box 5
Preventive treatment (taken daily to decrease frequency and severity of frequent headaches)

Antihypertensive medications: β-blockers (propranolol, atenolol), calcium-channel blocker (verapamil), angiotensin II receptor antagonist (candesartan)

Anticonvulsants: topiramate, gabapentin, valproate, zonisamide

Antidepressant medications: tricyclic antidepressants (nortriptyline, amitriptyline), selective serotonin reuptake inhibitors, selective serotonin/norepinephrine reuptake inhibitors

Nonsteroidal anti-inflammatory drugs: indomethacin, ibuprofen, naproxen

Supplements: riboflavin, magnesium, butterbur, Co-Q 10, feverfew

OnabotulinumtoxinA

Episodic Tension-Type Headache

A. At least 10 episodes of headache occurring on less than 1 day per month on average (<12 days per year) and fulfilling criteria B to D[5]
B. Lasting from 30 minutes to 7 days
C. At least 2 of the following 4 characteristics:
   1. Bilateral location
   2. Pressing or tightening (nonpulsating) quality
   3. Mild or moderate intensity
   4. Not aggravated by routine physical activity such as walking or climbing stairs
D. Both of the following:
   1. No nausea or vomiting
   2. No more than 1 of photophobia or phonophobia
E. Not better accounted for by another ICHD-3 diagnosis

The patient with occasional TTH will self-treat with over-the-counter pain medications, generally without involving medical consultation. NSAIDs and combination analgesics with caffeine are the most effective over-the-counter pain medications. However, once the headaches become more frequent than a couple of days per week, with concomitant increased use of acute pain medications, medication-overuse headache may occur and a preventive medication is indicated. Medication-overuse headache cannot be treated effectively until the offending acute pain medication has been discontinued. Lifestyle modifications used for migraine management are also used for prevention of TTH, with treatment of accompanying mood disorders or stressors. Preventive medications are also used to decrease the frequency and severity of chronic TTH, with tricyclic antidepressants generally being the most effective.[28]

CLUSTER HEADACHE AND OTHER TRIGEMINAL AUTONOMIC CEPHALALGIAS

A 42-year-old woman complained of left periorbital headaches. She had suffered headaches since childhood, with a family history of migraines. For about 3 years she noted severe pain around her left eye, occurring episodically for more than 10 days per month, lasting for 3 to 4 hours, accompanied by unilateral ptosis, pupillary dilatation, conjunctival redness, and tearing. Nausea accompanied these headaches, which were different from her usual migraine headaches. She also had chronic bilateral frontal pressure and a mild bilateral headache with menses. She was referred to an ophthalmologist who diagnosed migraines and suggested sodium valproate and sumatriptan, without relief. Brain imaging was normal. Headaches continued and she had to quit her job. On examination the patient had slightly increased left pupillary diameter. Indomethacin 75 mg, 1 a day for 2 weeks, then 2 a day, was suggested. When she increased the dose to 150 mg a day the left periorbital headaches disappeared completely for months, except for 2 mild headaches associated with significant stress.

TACs are one-sided, periorbital headaches with prominent cranial parasympathetic autonomic features, which are lateralized and ipsilateral to the headache (**Box 6**). Autonomic symptoms include conjunctival injection and/or lacrimation, nasal congestion and/or rhinorrhea, eyelid edema, forehead and facial sweating/flushing, and miosis and/or ptosis. Not all of these symptoms are present with all headaches. In contrast to patients with migraines, who tend to become quiet and withdrawn during attacks of severe pain, patients with TACs may be agitated, restless, or aggressive during the pain. The headaches are classified based on the duration and characteristics of the pain, and the response to the prescription NSAID indomethacin.[29]

Box 6
Trigeminal autonomic cephalalgias

Cluster headache

Paroxysmal hemicrania[a]

Short-lasting unilateral neuralgiform headache attacks

  Short-lasting unilateral neuralgiform headache attacks with conjunctival injection and tearing (SUNCT)

  Short-lasting unilateral neuralgiform headache attacks with cranial autonomic symptoms (SUNA)

Hemicrania continua[a]

  [a] Indomethacin-responsive headache.
  From Headache Classification Committee of the International Headache Society (IHS). The international classification of headache disorders, 3rd edition (beta version). Cephalalgia 2013;33:629–808; with permission.

Cluster headaches occur more often in middle-aged men, and may be associated with smoking and alcohol use. Cluster headaches tend to occur in the early morning hours, awakening the man from sleep with excruciating pain and autonomic symptoms. The attacks tend to occur daily for a period of weeks to months, and then remit for months to years. The attacks are relatively short in duration but the pain is very intense, and they are best treated with preventive medication, such as verapamil, steroids, and topiramate. Acute attacks may be treated with inhaled oxygen, subcutaneous sumatriptan injection, and nasal triptans. Cluster headaches characteristically are not responsive to indomethacin. Treatment of patients with cluster headaches often requires multiple acute and preventive medications at escalating doses, necessitating neurologic consultation. MRI to rule out an underlying mass lesion may be needed in patients with new onset of cluster-headache symptoms.

Other TACs have attacks with pain and associated symptoms similar to those of cluster headaches; but these headaches are shorter lasting, more frequent, and occur more commonly in females. Some TACs respond specifically to preventive treatment with indomethacin. Hemicrania continua is a persistent, generally side-locked unilateral headache type associated with ipsilateral autonomic symptoms that is, by definition, responsive to indomethacin. A continuous milder unilateral pain occurs at baseline, with a more severe superimposed unilateral facial pain of shorter duration. As noted in the case history described earlier, the eye findings include both miosis and mydriasis in these headaches that tend to be more common in women. In a study of 39 patients, only 8% had side-alternating pain. Of patients with hemicrania continua, 97% had at least 1 of the various cranial autonomic features during exacerbations: lacrimation (73%), nasal congestion (51%), conjunctival injection (46%) and ptosis (40%), facial flushing (40%), rhinorrhea, forehead/facial sweating, itching eye, eyelid edema, sense of aural fullness and periaural swelling, miosis, mydriasis, and swelling of the cheek and face. Migraine-like symptoms of phonophobia, photophobia, and motion sensitivity were common. About two-thirds of patients with severe hemicrania continua pain noted agitation and/or restlessness, and about one-quarter were aggressive, mainly verbally.[30]

Paroxysmal hemicranias are attacks of severe, strictly unilateral pain, which can be orbital, supraorbital, or temporal, lasting 2 to 30 minutes, and occurring several or many times a day. Both of these headache types are accompanied by ipsilateral autonomic symptoms, a characteristic of the other types of TACs. Both hemicrania continua and paroxysmal hemicranias respond to indomethacin used preventively at doses of 75 mg, increasing to 225 mg a day as needed or tolerated. A nonneurologist who recognizes the clinical description of these headaches should suggest a trial of increasing doses of indomethacin, often with a gratifying and diagnostic response to treatment. Should the headaches not respond to indomethacin as expected, imaging and referral to a neurologist are indicated.

Short-lasting unilateral neuralgiform headache attacks are short-lasting attacks of unilateral pain lasting 5 to 240 seconds, occurring from 3 to 200 times per day. The pain is stabbing or pulsating in an orbital, supraorbital, or temporal location. The attacks can be classified as short-lasting unilateral neuralgiform headache attacks with conjunctival injection and tearing (SUNCT), or short-lasting unilateral neuralgiform headache attacks with cranial autonomic symptoms (SUNA), depending on the type of accompanying autonomic symptoms. These headache types are particularly difficult to treat and do not respond to indomethacin. Patients with such headaches are best referred to a headache specialist for brain imaging and a trial of lamotrigine.

Patients with these uncommon primary headache types may present to an otolaryngologist for evaluation, especially as the unilateral facial pain with ipsilateral facial swelling and nasal symptoms may be interpreted as being related to sinus disease. Recognition of these headaches can lead to a specific and appropriate treatment. An otolaryngologist recognizing these headaches can initiate indomethacin treatment, often with a rapid and gratifying response. The drug's major side effect is gastric distress, which decreases if the medication is taken with meals or a proton-pump inhibitor. If the diagnosis of any side-locked headache is not clear, with or without significant autonomic symptoms, a trial of indomethacin at an increasing dose may be indicated. This NSAID, with a therapeutic response that is virtually diagnostic of hemicrania continua and paroxysmal hemicranias, can also be used to treat other headache types. Primary stabbing headache is a transient stabbing pain in the distribution of the first division of the trigeminal nerve, lasting seconds but occurring multiple times per day. Exertional headaches can be precipitated by exercise, cough, Valsalva, or orgasm, and are often specifically responsive to indomethacin.

SECONDARY HEADACHES

Headaches with persistent focal neurologic complaints, as distinct from symptoms that are clearly due to a migraine aura, should be evaluated by a neurologist. However, some headaches that may not be accompanied by focal neurologic complaints or findings on examination may still indicate an underlying neurologic disorder that needs immediate and specific neurologic treatment. A thunderclap headache is the sudden onset of severe headache pain without gradual buildup of pain. One of the most common causes of a sudden-onset headache is pain from a rapidly escalating migraine headache, primary cough headache, exertional headache, and orgasmic headache. Pain from subarachnoid hemorrhage, reversible cerebral vasospasm syndrome, cerebral venous thrombosis, and intracerebral hemorrhage may all present with sudden onset of pain without readily discernible neurologic defects. Obviously these patients with vascular causes of sudden-onset headache should be referred emergently for neurologic evaluation.

Although secondary headaches are generally treated from symptom onset by neurologists, patients with some secondary headaches may present initially to the otolaryngologist. Thrombosis of cerebral veins or venous sinuses may occur in the setting of oral contraceptives, head trauma, dehydration, infection, coagulation disorders, pregnancy, or cancer. Although patients with cerebral venous thrombosis generally present with headache or seizures, sudden unilateral sensorineural hearing loss, pulsatile tinnitus, or vertigo may be early and rare symptoms of this disorder.[31] Disorders of cerebrospinal fluid (CSF) dynamics can present with symptoms that may direct a patient to an otolaryngologist. Patients (generally obese women) with idiopathic intracranial hypertension may note pulsatile tinnitus as well as holocephalgic pain, transient visual obscurations, and sixth-nerve weakness. Immediate referral to a neurologist and an ophthalmologist is warranted because if left untreated this headache type, with increased CSF pressure, can result in visual loss from optic-nerve compression. Papilledema and elevated opening pressure on lumbar puncture, without any mass lesion on brain imaging, confirm the diagnosis. A headache resulting from decreased CSF pressure causes holocephalgic pain that is worse upright and improved recumbent, potentially interpreted as a sinus-related symptom. Severe sensorineural hearing loss with a headache has been described in spontaneous intracranial hypotension.[32] Leakage of CSF through a dural tear may result in enhancement of the leptomeninges on MRI of the brain in intracranial hypotension. Vascular lesions producing headache and pulsatile tinnitus include a dural arteriovenous fistula[33] and arterial dissection.[34]

SUMMARY

Patients with headaches consult with physicians in many different specialties; however, those who have an abnormal neurologic examination or red flags in their history should be referred for neurologic evaluation. A neurologist should also be consulted when the patient does not respond as expected to appropriate pain medications. Most patients who seek medical consultation for frequent headaches, without other neurologic symptoms and with a normal neurologic examination, have migraine headaches. Lifestyle modification and triptans used up to a few times per week are appropriate for most episodic migraine sufferers. Preventive medications, selected based on individual patient characteristics, are appropriate when the increased frequency and severity of migraines produces disability and impaired quality of life. Neurologic consultation may be indicated to help in the selection and dosing of preventive medications. Patients with unilateral side-locked headaches, without or with autonomic symptoms, should be treated with a trial of increasing dose of daily indomethacin to rule out indomethacin-responsive TACs, such as hemicrania continua or paroxysmal hemicranias.

REFERENCES

1. Farri A, Enrico A, Farri F. Headaches of otolaryngological interest: current status while awaiting revision of classification. Practical considerations and expectations. Acta Otorhinolaryngol Ital 2012;32:77–86.
2. Suarez P, Clark G. Oral conditions of 1,049 patients referred to a university-based oral medicine and orofacial pain center. Spec Care Dentist 2007;27:191–5.
3. Benoliel R, Eliav E. Primary headache disorders. Dent Clin North Am 2013;57: 513–39.
4. Alonso AA, Nixdorf DR. Case series of four different headache types presenting as tooth pain. J Endod 2006;32:1110–3.
5. Headache Classification Committee of the International Headache Society (IHS). The international classification of headache disorders, 3rd edition (beta version). Cephalalgia 2013;33:629–808.

6. Shapiro RE. Lagniappe: the impact of headache disorders in America. Headache 2013;53:196–204.
7. Reneman L, de Win MM, Booij J, et al. Incidental head and neck findings on MRI in young healthy volunteers: prevalence and clinical implications. AJNR Am J Neuroradiol 2012;33:1971–4.
8. Morris Z, Whiteley WN, Longstreth WT, et al. Incidental findings on brain magnetic resonance imaging: systematic review and meta-analysis. BMJ 2009;339:b3016.
9. Kruit MC, van Buchem MA, Launer LJ, et al. Migraine is associated with an increased risk of deep white matter lesions, subclinical posterior circulation infarcts and brain iron accumulation: the population-based MRI CAMERA study. Cephalalgia 2010;30:129–36.
10. Palm-Meinders IH, Koppen H, Terwindt GM, et al. Structural brain changes in migraine. JAMA 2012;308:1889–97.
11. Lester MS, Liu BP. Imaging in the evaluation of headache. Med Clin North Am 2013;97:243–65.
12. Wöber-Bingöl C. Epidemiology of migraine and headache in children and adolescents. Curr Pain Headache Rep 2013;17:341.
13. Brandes JL. Migraine in women. Continuum (Minneap Minn) 2012;18:835–52.
14. Furman JM, Marcus DA, Balaban CD. Vestibular migraine: clinical aspects and pathophysiology. Lancet Neurol 2013;12:706–15.
15. Neuhauser H, Lempert T. Vestibular migraine. Neurol Clin 2009;27:379–91.
16. Mikulec AA, Faraji F, Kinsella LJ. Evaluation of the efficacy of caffeine cessation, nortriptyline, and topiramate therapy in vestibular migraine and complex dizziness of unknown etiology. Am J Otolaryngol 2012;33:121–7.
17. Diener HC, Kurth T, Dodick D. Patent foramen ovale, stroke, and cardiovascular disease in migraine. Curr Opin Neurol 2007;20:310–9.
18. Davis D, Gregson J, Willeit P, et al. Patent foramen ovale, ischemic stroke and migraine: systematic review and stratified meta-analysis of association studies. Neuroepidemiology 2013;40:56–67.
19. Loder E. Triptan therapy in migraine. N Engl J Med 2010;363:63–70.
20. Kari E, DelGaudio JM. Treatment of sinus headache as migraine: the diagnostic utility of triptans. Laryngoscope 2008;118:2235–9.
21. Langer-Gould AM, Anderson WE, Armstrong MJ, et al. The American Academy of Neurology's Top Five Choosing Wisely recommendations. Neurology 2013; 81(11):1004–11.
22. Tepper SJ. Opioids should not be used in migraine. Headache 2012;52(Suppl 1): 30–4.
23. Abrams BM. Medication overuse headaches. Med Clin North Am 2013;97: 337–52.
24. Tepper SJ. Medication-overuse headache. Continuum (Minneap Minn) 2012;18: 807–22.
25. Silberstein SD, Holland S, Freitag F, et al. Evidence-based guideline update: pharmacologic treatment for episodic migraine prevention in adults: report of the Quality Standards Subcommittee of the American Academy of Neurology and the American Headache Society. Neurology 2012;78:1337–45.
26. Kamyar M, Varner M. Epilepsy in pregnancy. Clin Obstet Gynecol 2013;56: 330–41.
27. Holland S, Silberstein SD, Freitag F, et al. Evidence-based guideline update: NSAIDs and other complementary treatments for episodic migraine prevention in adults: report of the Quality Standards Subcommittee of the American Academy of Neurology and the American Headache Society. Neurology 2012;78:1346–53.

28. Bendtsen L, Bigal ME, Cerbo R, et al. Guidelines for controlled trials of drugs in tension-type headache: second edition. Cephalalgia 2010;30:1–16.
29. Goadsby PJ. Trigeminal autonomic cephalalgias. Continuum (Minneap Minn) 2012;18:883–95.
30. Cittadini E, Goadsby PJ. Hemicrania continua: a clinical study of 39 patients with diagnostic implications. Brain 2010;133:1973–86.
31. Braun EM, Stanzenberger H, Nemetz U, et al. Sudden unilateral hearing loss as first sign of cerebral sinus venous thrombosis? A 3-year retrospective analysis. Otol Neurotol 2013;34:657–61.
32. Chen S, Hagiwara M, Roehm PC. Spontaneous intracranial hypotension presenting with severe sensorineural hearing loss and headache. Otol Neurotol 2012;33: e65–6.
33. Choi JW, Kim BM, Kim DJ, et al. Hypoglossal canal dural arteriovenous fistula: incidence and the relationship between symptoms and drainage pattern. J Neurosurg 2013;119(4):955–60.
34. von Babo M, De Marchis GM, Sarikaya H, et al. Differences and similarities between spontaneous dissections of the internal carotid artery and the vertebral artery. Stroke 2013;44:1537–42.

What Do We Know About Rhinogenic Headache?

The Otolaryngologist's Challenge

Mark E. Mehle, MD[a,b,]*
Curtis P. Schreiber, MD

WITH AFTERWORD TO THE OTOLARYNGOLOGIST'S CHALLENGE: THE DIFFERENTIAL DIAGNOSIS OF THE POSITIVE SCAN BY CURTIS P. SCHREIBER

KEYWORDS

- Sinus headache • Rhinogenic headache • Contact point headache
- Migraine headache • Nasal pain

KEY POINTS

- Relatively few patients presenting with "sinus headache" complaints are found to have rhinogenic headache.
- Potential underlying causes of rhinogenic headache include acute rhinosinusitis, chronic rhinosinusitis, or mucosal contact point, with or without concha bullosa of the middle turbinate.
- Of these potential causes for rhinogenic headache, only acute rhinosinusitis is considered validated in the headache literature; the others remain controversial, although recent studies have supported chronic sinusitis as a potential cause of headache.
- The surgical literature regarding intranasal contact point intervention is enthusiastic but unscientific, and randomized, controlled studies are still needed in this contentious area.

Rhinogenic headache is a term that has been used in a variety of ways in the medical literature. Traditionally, it was used interchangeably with "sinus headache" until a wealth of literature showed that sinus headache complaints are likely to represent migraine and seldom represent a sinus infection.[1,2] The most recent (2013) *International Classification of Headache Disorders* by the International Headache Society (IHS) includes a category of secondary headaches, which, in turn, includes headache attributed to acute rhinosinusitis (**Box 1**), with the stipulation that other signs and symptoms of acute sinusitis are present. Chronic rhinosinusitis (CRS) is also supported as a cause of headache (**Box 2**) although some controversy still exists in this regard.

Disclosures: Speaker Bureau, Teva, Sunovion; Advisory Board, Merck, Teva, Sunovion.
[a] Northeast Ohio Medical University, 4209 Ohio 44, Rootstown, OH 44272, USA; [b] Private Practice, ENT and Allergy Health Services, 25761 Lorain Road, 3rd Floor, North Olmsted, OH 44070, USA
* Private Practice, ENT and Allergy Health Services, 25761 Lorain Road, 3rd Floor, North Olmsted, OH 44070.
E-mail address: Dr.m.mehle@att.net

Otolaryngol Clin N Am 47 (2014) 255–268
http://dx.doi.org/10.1016/j.otc.2013.10.006
0030-6665/14/$ – see front matter © 2014 Elsevier Inc. All rights reserved.

Box 1
Headache attributed to acute rhinosinusitis

Description:

Headache caused by acute rhinosinusitis and associated with other symptoms or clinical signs of this disorder.

Diagnostic criteria:

A. Any headache fulfilling criterion C

B. Clinical, nasal endoscopic, or imaging evidence of acute rhinosinusitis

C. Evidence of causation shown by at least 2 of the following:

    1. Headache has developed in temporal relation to the onset of the rhinosinusitis

    2. Either or both of the following:

        a. Headache has significantly worsened in parallel with worsening of the rhinosinusitis

        b. Headache has significantly improved or resolved in parallel with improvement in or resolution of the rhinosinusitis

    3. Headache is exacerbated by pressure applied over the paranasal sinuses

    4. In the case of a unilateral rhinosinusitis, headache is localized ipsilateral to it

D. Not better accounted for by another *International Classification of Headache Disorders, Third Edition* diagnosis

From Headache Classification Subcommittee of the International Headache Society. The International Classification of Headache Disorders, 3rd edition (beta version). Cephalalgia 2013;33:764; with permission.

Box 2
Headache attributed to chronic or recurring rhinosinusitis

Description:

Headache caused by a chronic infectious or inflammatory disorder of the paranasal sinuses and associated with other symptoms or clinical signs of the disorder.

Diagnostic criteria:

A. Any headache fulfilling criterion C

B. Clinical, nasal endoscopic, or imaging evidence of current or past infection or other inflammatory process within the paranasal sinuses

C. Evidence of causation shown by at least 2 of the following:

    1. Headache has developed in temporal relation to the onset of CRS

    2. Headache waxes and wanes in parallel with the degree of sinus congestion, drainage, and other symptoms of CRS

    3. Headache is exacerbated by pressure applied over the paranasal sinuses

    4. In the case of a unilateral rhinosinusitis, headache is localized ipsilateral to it

D. Not better accounted for by another *International Classification of Headache Disorders, Third Edition* diagnosis

Comment:

It has been controversial whether or not chronic sinus disease can produce persistent headache. Recent studies seem to support such causation.

From Headache Classification Subcommittee of the International Headache Society. The International Classification of Headache Disorders, 3rd edition (beta version). Cephalalgia 2013;33:765; with permission.

Headache attributed to disorder of the nasal mucosa, turbinates, or septum (**Box 3**) is described in the appendix of the *Classification*, although the questionable validity of this entity is noted.[3] This category replaced the term mucosal contact point headache, which was included in the appendix of the second edition *Classification* in 2004 and which has now been abandoned. This term is still used extensively in the surgical literature and is discussed in detail later.

Reviewing the literature on nonneoplastic rhinogenic headache is complicated by many factors: crossover symptoms with primary headache syndromes (especially migraine), published literature of surgical series lacking controls or precise inclusion or diagnostic criteria, and comorbidity between primary headaches and nasal diseases such as allergic rhinitis and CRS. Radiographic studies similarly have been less than reliable for inclusion or exclusion of rhinogenic headache. All of these factors make a review of this topic worthy of inclusion in this issue. Please note that neoplastic causes of nasal pain (eg, sinonasal carcinoma) are excluded in this discussion.

RELEVANT NASAL ANATOMY

The maxillary (V-2) and ophthalmic (V-1) divisions of the trigeminal nerve provide sensation to the nose and paranasal sinuses. These afferents project via the trigeminal ganglion to the trigeminal brainstem sensory nuclear complex (VBSNC). Autonomic innervation of the nose is provided by sympathetic nerve fibers (originating at the superior cervical ganglion, to the deep petrosal nerve, to the vidian nerve, then through the sphenopalatine ganglion) and parasympathetic fibers (from the superior salivatory nucleus of VII, then to the greater superficial petrosal nerve, vidian nerve, and synapsing then in the sphenopalatine ganglion). The trigeminal fibers in the nose terminate as bare nerve terminal endings, along with the parasympathetic nerves near the basal

---

Box 3
Headache attributed to disorder of the nasal mucosa, turbinates, or septum

Diagnostic criteria:

A. Any headache fulfilling criterion C

B. Clinical, nasal endoscopic, or imaging evidence of a hypertrophic or inflammatory process within the nasal cavity[a]

C. Evidence of causation shown by at least 2 of the following:

   1. Headache has developed in temporal relation to the onset of the intranasal lesion

   2. Headache has significantly improved or significantly worsened in parallel with improvement in (with or without treatment) or worsening of the nasal lesion

   3. Headache has significantly improved after local anesthesia of the mucosa in the region of the lesion

   4. Headache is ipsilateral to the site of the lesion

D. Not better accounted for by another *International Classification of Headache Disorders, Third Edition* diagnosis

   [a] Examples are concha bullosa and nasal septal spur.

From Headache Classification Subcommittee of the International Headache Society. The International Classification of Headache Disorders, 3rd edition (beta version). Cephalalgia 2013;33:804; with permission.

cells of the nasal epithelium. Unlike the skin or tendons, no specialized sensory organs are present.[4–6]

RELEVANT NEUROPHYSIOLOGY

Nasal pain is mediated by Aδ fibers (fast responding, primarily mechanoreceptive pain fibers) and C fibers (slower, unmyelinated fibers associated with a more dull pain from mechanothermal and chemosensory stimulation). Activation of the pain fibers is typified by the release of tachykinins (substance P, neurokinin A, neuropeptide K) and neuropeptides like calcitonin gene-related peptide. Sympathetic neurons are associated with neuropeptide Y, in addition to norepinephrine, and the parasympathetic fibers release acetylcholine and vasoactive intestinal peptide.[6–8] These neurotransmitters and neurochemicals are nonspecific markers of nerve activation and are associated with primary headache phenomena like migraine and seemingly unrelated disease such as allergic rhinitis, as well as rhinogenic pain.[9–11] Thus, earlier reports citing the presence of these chemicals (eg, substance P) as evidence for contact point headache validity were poorly founded.

Neuroplasticity is also a phenomenon of unclear cause, in which acute pain may become chronic or more easily triggered (hyperalgesia) or is temporarily reduced, with a temporary reduction of headache pain mediated by the VBSNC after induction of surgical pain in the same distribution.[6] This area of the brainstem (including the trigeminal nucleus caudalis) is critically important in the pathophysiology of migraine, as is covered elsewhere in this issue.

RELEVANT PSYCHOBIOLOGY

Researchers have documented the importance of cognitive dissonance as a factor in a possible placebo effect in surgical studies for headache. This effect stems from the fact that a patient reports a psychological benefit from a surgical procedure (which required pain or expense, initiated by the patients' willingness to participate) regardless if the surgery had no benefit (hence the dissonance between reality and psychological benefit).[12] This finding may thus confound studies evaluating surgical interventions for mucosal contact point or migraine surgeries.

PRIMARY HEADACHES AND RHINOGENIC HEADACHE

Most patients complaining of "sinus headache" have migraine as an underlying cause.[1,2,13,14] The pathophysiology of migraine has relevance to the topic of rhinogenic headache. Although the central nervous system is likely the initiator of the migraine process, this is followed by sensitization of the peripheral neurons of the trigeminal nerve. This situation can then lead to central sensitization at the level of the trigeminal nucleus caudalis in the brainstem, and pain in the distribution of the first (ophthalmic, V-1) or second (maxillary, V-2) divisions of the trigeminal nerve. This early sensitization phase is commonly accompanied by cutaneous allodynia (pain associated with ordinarily minor stimuli) in most patients (80%). The causation of pain by stimulation that is normally nonpainful often occurs in the distribution of V-1 and V-2.[15] This situation may include stimuli to the nose, such as breathing cold air. To make matters more complex, the migraine attack itself may include secondary nasal symptoms (possibly mediated from stimulation of the parasympathetic nervous system, via the superior salivatory nucleus of the seventh cranial nerve

[VII]).[1] Nasal engorgement could then lead to mucosal contact in areas of nasal narrowing with or without allodynia-related pain. This factor has been suggested as supporting a potentially beneficial role for contact point surgery, even in patients with underlying migraine.[16] Conversely, this situation may theoretically create a false-positive contact point test, in which application of an anesthetic or induction of pain (injection) in the nose may downregulate a migraine headache by interrupting a source of allodynia.

THE PROBLEM OF COMORBIDITY

Migraine is a common phenomenon, and does not exist in a vacuum. Jackson and Dial[17] reported that 49 of 100 patients referred to an ear, nose, and throat (ENT) office for sinus headache had migraine, but only 13% had migraine alone; 19 (of the migraineurs) had allergic rhinitis as well, 11 had sinusitis, and 6 had both allergic rhinitis and sinusitis. A second study[14] found extensive radiographic abnormalities on sinus computed tomography (CT) studies in patients with sinus headache with migraine. The mean CT scan Lund-Mackay (L-M) score in this study did not differ significantly between the migraine (2.1) and nonmigraine cohort (2.7). Five of the migraine group had substantial sinus disease radiographically (with L-M scores $\geq$5), as did 2 of the nonmigraineurs. A more recent study[18] found a history of headache in general to be more common in patients with CRS than in non-CRS controls, although a second series found that facial pain (not facial pressure), headache, and photophobia were negatively predictive of the presence of radiographic evidence of CRS.[19] CRS has been reported to be a factor in the worsening of the course of migraine, potentially making it more refractory or chronic.[20] Thus, the association of CRS and migraine remains unclear.

Allergic rhinitis and migraine have been found to be comorbid as well, with some evidence suggesting that allergy management may have some headache benefits in patients with both disorders.[9,21,22] Whether this situation stems from shared pathophysiology, reduction of mucosal contact, or perhaps from secondary benefits such as stress reduction in the migraineur remains to be seen.

RHINOGENIC HEADACHES

Strictly rhinogenic headaches are headaches that have their primary pathophysiology centered in the nose and have headache or facial pain as a secondary effect. The term sinus headache should be used to describe a patient complaint and does not accurately describe any underlying pathologic process.

Headache Attributed to Acute Rhinosinusitis

The clearest example of a rhinogenic headache is the headache associated with acute rhinosinusitis, and the criteria for this diagnosis are presented in **Box 1**. The supportive signs of acute sinusitis in the IHS publication closely mirror the diagnostic criteria for acute sinusitis published in the otolaryngology literature, focusing on congestion, purulent drainage, and anosmia/hyposmia as well as pressure or pain.[3,23]

CRS

The 2013 IHS *Classification* has validated chronic sinusitis as a cause of headache. Several studies have looked at headache as a symptom of CRS. Most of these studies did not use the IHS migraine criteria in assessing these headaches, which may have led to more robust conclusions regarding the role of CRS in these headaches as a cause of pain as opposed to a comorbid condition. In 2007, Clifton and Jones[24] found that 29% of patients with CRS complained of facial pain and that more than 60% seemed to respond to medical therapy. Several studies have shown substantial improvement in headache symptoms with functional endoscopic sinus surgery (FESS) for CRS, although other recent series have failed to show a benefit. In the report of Soler and colleagues[25] in 2008, headache was described as the most disabling symptom in 29% of a series of patients with CRS undergoing FESS, but no evidence of postoperative headache improvement was found. Chester and colleagues[26] in 2009 published a meta-analysis of published series of FESS patients with CRS, and found that among all of the symptoms analyzed, all of the scores improved postoperatively, but headache scores improved the least.

MUCOSAL CONTACT POINT HEADACHE

Sluder (1908) described a syndrome of recurrent hemifacial/hemicranial pain with concomitant parasympathetic symptoms (unilateral rhinorrhea and congestion). This headache type was later associated with contact point neuralgia, although the original description did not stipulate associated anatomic anomalies.[27,28] Recent publications have associated these symptoms with a cluster headache variant.[27]

Sinus pain was further studied by Wolff (1948)[29] with a series of experiments directly manipulating various areas of the sinonasal mucosa and reporting the sensitivity as well as the patterns of referred pain. This investigator found that the sinus ostia were more sensitive than the sinus cavities and that the turbinates seemed more sensitive than the septal mucosa. The pain radiation patterns reported in these studies have been frequently cited over the years, although recent work has questioned the accuracy of the findings. Abu-Bakra and Jones,[30] for example, found that neither local pressure in the nose nor the application of substance P to various points in the nose in 10 volunteers produced referred pain to the face or headache.

Radiographically, contact points are common on sinus CT scans but correlate poorly with facial pain or headache. In a study of 973 patients referred for a sinus CT scan, the incidence of radiographic contact points was 4%, and did not differ among those patients with facial pain complaints (42% of the patients) and those who were pain free. Moreover, in patients with unilateral facial pain, the contact point was on the opposite side in 50%.[31] Other studies have shown a higher incidence of contact points (up to 55%), but even in these studies, there was no clear correlation to the presence or absence of pain.[32]

A study from 2009[33] noted no association between CT findings and outcomes of minimally invasive endoscopic sinus surgeries conducted for rhinogenic headaches, despite using radiographic criteria such as contact points and concha bullosa as inclusion criteria for surgery. This particular study reported a surgical success rate (reduction of headache frequency, duration, or intensity) of 84.8% (28 of 33 patients). A mean follow-up of more than 18 months was reported. All of the failures had clear septal spurs, and no association was noted between contact points and surgical outcomes.

In addition to contact points, middle turbinate pneumatization (ie, concha bullosa) has been incriminated in the cause of headache. Concha bullosa may be found in up to 50% of middle turbinates.[34,35] Goldsmith and colleagues[34] reported their experience with middle turbinate headache syndrome, noting that contact with adjacent mucosa (with or without concha bullosa) was present in these patients. All patients had headaches lacking an aura, and no response to ergotamine therapy. These investigators reported that 6 of 6 patients improved with middle turbinate surgery, which included FESS and septoplasty if it was believed to be indicated. Two improved with medical management alone. Like many studies on this topic, there was no randomization or control group and no screening for migraine headache, and follow-up was variable. Other studies have failed to find an association between concha bullosa and sidedness of headaches.[14]

Kunachak (2002)[36] reported successful headache resolution in patients undergoing in-office middle turbinate lateralization. These 55 patients all had headache of endo-scopically proven origin based on anatomic findings and response to topical lidocaine. All had complete responses reported in a follow-up of 6 to 84 months, although 7 of them (13%) required a second procedure. Migraine was not discussed in this study.

An Italian study[37] presented a series of 26 patients who had headaches that improved with partial resection of a pneumatized middle turbinate. These patients all had a normal neurologic examination, but no mention was made of migraine screening. All patients were reported to have pain on palpation of the superior and medial orbital rim (Ewing and Grunwald points, respectively), which was described by the investigators as confirming pain that was clearly of secondary origin. No randomization or controls were used, and patients were followed for 180 days.

Despite poor anatomic correlation, contact points have been the focus of surgical intervention for sinus headache complaints. Part of this support stems from the use of office anesthetic testing to support the role of the contact point in triggering the headaches in question. In the Goldsmith study cited earlier, cocaine was used to anesthetize the contact point in question, with a positive response (ie, resolution of an active headache) being used to support surgical intervention in medical failures.[34] Similar testing has been suggested using injected lidocaine, or topical anesthetics of various kinds in an effort to abort headaches. Using a topical anesthetic, Ramadan[38] found no correlation between a positive test in the office and improvement of headache after surgical contact point resection, citing an approximately 60% improvement either way. Similarly, Abu-Samra and colleagues[39] (see later discussion) found no correlation between a positive local anesthetic test and patient satisfaction after contact point surgery, although in their series a complete response to surgery was significantly more common in anesthetic responders. Despite poor clinical correlation, the IHS guidelines for the diagnosis of headache attributed to disorder of the nasal mucosa, turbinates, or septum support this test, regardless of validity.

Abu-Samra and colleagues[39] in 2011 published a series of 42 patients who underwent septoplasty with or without endoscopic partial turbinectomy for contact point headaches and chronic daily headache, in the presence of chronic migraine (20 patients) or chronic tension-type headache (22) using IHS criteria. These patients were followed a minimum of 1 year postoperatively, and the mean headache days per month was reduced from 22 to 7.

In 2011, Bektas and colleagues[40] published a series of 36 patients with rhinogenic contact point headaches and reported that all patients had a reduction of postoperative headache or intensity of pain during headaches, with 19 (52.7%) reporting a complete absence of headache pain. The surgeries performed included septoplasty, anterior ethmoidectomy, partial turbinectomy, and septal spur resection, in varying combinations. All patients had failed neurologic therapy as well as a topical nasal steroid trial and had confirmatory anatomic findings on CT scan or endoscopically, although no mention was made as to whether the headaches were migrainous. Minimum follow-up in this study was 6 months.

Taken as a whole, the literature regarding mucosal contact point surgery is questionably supportive of a role for surgery in some patients but suffers from poor or inconsistent diagnostic/inclusion criteria, surgical technique used, concomitant comorbidity (primary headache or otherwise), and inconsistent follow-up. None of the studies available is truly randomized or blinded, and all are level 4 evidence by evidence-based medicine criteria.[41,42] A summary of outcomes of some recent studies is included in **Table 1**. Neuroplasticity and cognitive dissonance may explain the improvement reported in these surgical patients, as emphasized by Jones and colleagues.[42] The partial responses reported in many series also support the notion that the headache complaints are multifactorial in many patients. Two recent literature reviews came to similar conclusions: randomized, controlled studies are needed to determine with any scientific accuracy whether contact point resection is beneficial to the patient with facial pain/headache, and that surgery should be considered an option only after extensive medical workup and management.[41,42]

SURGERY FOR MIGRAINE RELIEF?

There have been reports in the ENT and headache literature that migraineurs with mucosal contact point may benefit from resection of these areas. Behin and colleagues[16] and Abu-Samra and colleagues[39] have independently reported series of contact point patients with documented migraine, in which a positive benefit was reported after contact point surgery in most patients. This finding supports several reports in the plastic surgery literature by Guyuron and colleagues[43,44] that intranasal surgery may provide a benefit to migraine sufferers unresponsive to medications,[45] but all of these reports suffer from the same drawbacks mentioned earlier for contact point surgery in general. Whether these interventions are taking advantage of placebo responses, neuroplasticity, or other unknown mechanisms remains to be seen.

Guyuron and colleagues[44] (2011) reviewed their 5-year outcomes for surgical intervention in migraine sufferers and reported that 61 (88%) of 69 patients who underwent surgical intervention of 1 or more migraine trigger sites had a positive response (reduction of the frequency, duration, and intensity of headache), with 20 (29%) reporting a complete absence of migraine headaches. Among these patients, 52 of the 69 underwent septoplasty or partial turbinectomy, but only 3 underwent nasal surgery alone (the others also had neurolysis of cutaneous branches of the trigeminal facial or occipital nerves, or muscle resection in adjacent areas).

Table 1
Surgical intervention for apparent nasal contact point rhinogenic headache: a sample of the literature published in recent years

Author, Year	Outcome Reported
Novak & Makek,[47] 1992	78.5% complete response, benefit in all patients (n = 299)
Sindwani & Wright,[48] 2003	54% cured, another 38.5% better; only 1 failure (n = 13)
Behin et al,[16] 2006	92% improved (n = 21)
Mokbel et al,[49] 2010	61.66% symptom free, 19.2% no better (n = 120)
Bektas et al,[40] 2011	57% complete relief, all better (n = 36)
Mohebbi et al,[50] 2010	83% better, 11% cured (n = 36)
Yazici et al,[46] 2010	Surgical patients (n = 38) had a significant reduction of headache symptoms based on visual analogue scale
Abu-Samra et al,[39] 2011	19% totally headache free, 62% improved (n = 42)

Data from Refs.[16,39,40,46–50]

In a more recent publication[45] of the Guyuron migraine surgery series, it was noted that patients with nasal triggers alone had a 50% success rate in headache improvement (3 of 6 patients), lower than the series as a whole, in which botulinum type A therapy response was a prognosticator of a favorable surgical outcome (90.3% favorable response to surgery vs 72.3% for botulinum nonresponders). The migraineurs with nasal triggers alone had poor correlation between a botulinum response and surgical response.

In 2010, Yazici and colleagues[46] performed rhinologic evaluations in 99 patients with primary headache, 70 of whom had migraine. Seventy-three of the 99 were found to have nasal abnormalities, consisting of septal deviation, turbinate hypertrophy, contact points, and concha bullosa. Fifty-three patients of 99 were described as not responding to medical therapy, and 38 of these underwent nasal surgery. Headache severity based on visual analogue scales 3 and 6 months after surgery was significantly reduced.

PATIENT MANAGEMENT

When a patient presents with sinus headache, knowledge of potential rhinogenic sources makes the otolaryngologist a key component of the management team. Regardless of initial impressions, the following steps in workup are of key importance:

1. A thorough history is of the greatest importance to the diagnosing physician or practitioner. The nature, intensity, duration, and presentation are keys to primary headache diagnosis. Every otolaryngologist should be familiar with the IHS diagnostic criteria for migraine (covered elsewhere in this issue) and have a good working relation with a neurologist who has an interest in headache. Even in an otolaryngology office, most patients with sinus headache are found to have migraine. Family history is also of importance, because many migraineurs have a strong family history of this disorder.
2. Medication history is also of great importance. Many patients have a long history of unsuccessful management of their headache with rhinitis medications or antibiotics. Others may have extensive use of over-the-counter (OTC) medication use. The phenomenon of chronic daily headache may have an association with OTC analgesic overuse.[3] Caffeine has long been associated with exacerbating the course of migraine headaches; the author has seen a similar pattern with the abuse of OTC sympathomimetic decongestants like pseudoephedrine.
3. Physical examination should include a thorough otolaryngologic examination to look for extranasal sources of pain (eg, temporomandibular joint problems, covered elsewhere in this issue) as well as intranasal disease. The presence of anatomic variants such as a mucosal contact point or a concha bullosa of the middle turbinate is not diagnostic of a rhinogenic headache syndrome; most of these are asymptomatic. Moreover, a response to a topical anesthetic during a headache (ie, headache resolution) does not confirm this syndrome, either (see earlier discussion). A false-positive may theoretically be seen in some migraineurs, via allodynia resolution or neuroplasticity.
4. Radiographic studies may be reasonable if the diagnosis is unclear or if physical findings are supportive of the need for further workup. It is reasonable to consider these studies in any patient on whom surgery is contemplated for headache. Positive radiographic findings are not diagnostic of rhinogenic headache and may have little correlation to clinical presentations.

5. Medical management is the mainstay of headache treatment. Migraine management is particularly helpful and should be pursued exhaustively before consideration of any surgical intervention. This topic is covered elsewhere, but is key in surgical decision making; surgery is always a last resort regardless of physical or radiographic findings.
6. Surgical management is a last resort based on the preceding discussion. Any discussion of rhinogenic headache surgery with patients should include the fact that these surgeries are poorly supported scientifically and that failures are common. Regardless, surgery can be considered an option in these patients, based on a review of the literature.

SUMMARY

The literature regarding rhinogenic headache remains promising but inconclusive. It is important for the practitioner to realize that sinus headache complaints and rhinogenic headache are 2 different entities: the former is a patient presentation, which is frequently found to represent migraine, and the latter is a concept in which nasal or paranasal sinus disease is believed to be responsible for facial or head pain. Excluding neoplastic processes, the clearest example of rhinogenic headache is the headache associated with acute rhinosinusitis. This cause is clearly supported by the otolaryngologic and neurologic literature, but headache alone is a poor predictor of rhinosinusitis. Chronic sinusitis remains a possible source of headache, but mucosal contact point as a source of headache remains contentious, despite an enthusiastic but largely unscientific body of literature supporting it. The association between migraine headache and concomitant sinonasal disease is also in need of elucidation, because there may be significant benefit from the management of comorbid conditions in these patients. Clearly, randomized, controlled trials would be the ideal next step toward furthering our understanding of these important issues.

AFTERWORD – The Otolaryngologist's Challenge: The Differential Diagnosis of the Positive Scan

Curtis P. Schreiber, MD
Neurologist and Headache Specialist in Private Practice, Citizens Memorial Healthcare, Bolivar, MO, USA

As advanced imaging became available and the technology progressed to provide more and more highly detailed images of the nervous system, it was often joked that the role of the neurologist would become diminished and relegated to providing a differential diagnosis for the negative scan. Obviously, this dire prediction for neurology never came to fruition. In rhinogenic headache, the tables have clearly been turned, and the challenge for the otolaryngologist has become that of providing a differential diagnosis for a positive scan.

Our patients' perceptions can often lead the diagnostic evaluation. As Dr Mehle wisely points out, the term sinus headache should really be reserved to describe a symptom and not a pain mechanism. For a patient, any head pain that occurs in the frontal or maxillary regions might have the convincing feel of sinus discomfort and therefore may be interpreted as originating from the underlying sinuses. This issue was brilliantly illustrated to me when we recruited a small study of patients with both sinus headache and diagnosed migraine. A well-educated woman presented for the study who had been diagnosed with migraine by her medical care provider and who had an effective treatment plan for her migraines. She also had self-diagnosed sinus headaches, which were not responding to her over-the-counter sinus medication treatment regimen. For our study, we needed to be sure that the patients were able to differentiate their headache types at the onset of the headache attack. This patient reported that it was easy for her to determine which type of headache was occurring. Her main differentiating feature was that before her sinus headache she had sparkling lights in her peripheral vision. Despite what is obvious to the clinician, that she was having a migraine aura, she knew that the headache that followed the sparkling lights was a sinus headache, because it centered in the frontal area and she had mild nasal congestion. She never even thought of treating her sinus headache with her migraine-specific medication and continued to do poorly with her management of these headaches. The headaches that she identified as migraine did not have a visual aura and responded nicely to her prescribed migraine medication.

Another significant issue that we all face when evaluating patients with headaches is the reliance on imaging by the medical community and the expectation of patients that imaging is required for accurate diagnosis. In a busy primary care office, an order for an imaging procedure may be more quickly offered than a thorough history and physical examination. An abnormal scan report may prompt a referral to a specialist rather than a recheck with the primary care provider. It is also true that patients often not only expect, but often demand, imaging procedures for their complaints. When something is found on the imaging study, they expect a specialist to provide consultation and definitive treatment. As Dr Mehle's review has pointed out, abnormal findings on scans do not always implicate a pathophysiologic mechanism. Similar issues are commonly seen as a result of the prevalence of radiographic evidence for spinal disease in patients without back pain and Arnold-Chiari malformation in patients without headache.

Our professional societies are trying to provide us with a better framework for understanding these patients and to give us better guidance in their management. This guidance is clearly a work in progress. As Dr Mehle has pointed out, the headache bible, the International Classification of Headache Disorders by the International Headache Society (IHS), is a work in progress. This work is progressing, but at an agonizingly slow pace. The third and most recent revision (2013) took 9 years for the expert panel to finalize after the second revision appeared in 2004. Although these criteria are the current gold standard for headache diagnosis, they are clearly a work in progress and will evolve as our understanding of the headache patient progresses. The acceptance of structural disease as the cause has long been contentious in the headache field, and its incorporation in the appendix ("Headaches attributed to disorders of the nasal mucosa, turbinates or septum") rather than in the main classification system indicates that this is still a work in progress and has not been completely adopted. Although the IHS criteria are a useful classification system and are widely accepted as a way to find a reasonably homogeneous group of patients for research studies, it has had poor penetration into the daily practice of primary care clinicians. As specialists on the receiving end of the headache patient referral, it is our responsibility to apply our knowledge of the patient, their history and physical examination, and our review of their imaging findings as we establish a diagnosis and recommend a treatment plan. Having a working knowledge of the current diagnostic criteria for the commonly seen headache types certainly aids in our diagnostic approach.

So where does this leave the otolaryngologist? Often, the otolaryngologist is in the position of considering the differential diagnosis of the positive scan. I recommend that if you have made it to this point of this article, you go back to the end of Dr Mehle's article and reread the section on patient management. His is a well-considered and practical approach for evaluating patients with the symptom of sinus headaches. Maximal medical management should be required before consideration of surgical intervention. You need to consider the medical management that the patient has undertaken before considering surgery. Did they have adequate trial of at least 2 headache preventive medications? Did they modify factors that could potentially worsen headache (eg, eliminate caffeine and overuse of analgesics)? If appropriate, did they have an adequate trial of migraine-specific medications for the headache attacks? Not all neurologists have an interest in headache, and not all clinicians who provide excellent headache care are neurologists. You may need to make the referral forward to a headache specialist rather than sending the patient directly back to the originator of the referral. The otolaryngologist can play a pivotal role in improved patient care, even when a positive scan is really negative.

REFERENCES

1. Schreiber CP, Hutchinson S, Webster CJ, et al. Prevalence of migraine in patients with a history of self-reported or physician-diagnosed "sinus" headache. Arch Intern Med 2004;164:1769–72.
2. Mehle ME, Schreiber C. Sinus headache, migraine, and the otolaryngologist. Otolaryngol Head Neck Surg 2005;133:489–96.
3. Headache Classification Subcommittee of the International Headache Society. The International Classification of Headache Disorders, 3rd edition (beta version). Cephalalgia 2013;33:629–808.
4. Paff GH. Anatomy of the head and neck. Philadelphia: WB Saunders; 1973.
5. Hollinshead WH. Anatomy for surgeons: the head and neck. Philadelphia: Harper and Row; 1982.
6. Sessle BJ. Acute and chronic craniofacial pain: brainstem mechanisms of nociceptive transmission and neuroplasticity, and their clinical correlates. Crit Rev Oral Biol Med 2000;11:57–91.
7. Baraniuk JN. Neurogenic mechanisms in rhinosinusitis. Curr Allergy Asthma Rep 2001;1:252–61.
8. Baraniuk JN, Lundgren JD, Okayama M, et al. Substance P and neurokinin A in human nasal mucosa. Am J Respir Cell Mol Biol 1991;4:228–36.
9. Mehle ME. Migraine and allergy: a review and clinical update. Curr Allergy Asthma Rep 2012;12(3):240–5. http://dx.doi.org/10.1007/s11882-012-0251-x.
10. Bellamy J, Cady R, Durham P. Salivary levels of CGRP and VIP in rhinosinusitis and migraine patients. Headache 2006;46:24–33.
11. Gelfand EW. Inflammatory mediators in allergic rhinitis. J Allergy Clin Immunol 2004;114:S135–8.
12. Homer JJ, Sheard CE, Jones NS. Cognitive dissonance, the placebo effect and the evaluation of surgical results. Clin Otolaryngol 2000;25:195–9.
13. Eross E, Dodick D, Eross M. The sinus, allergy and migraine study. Headache 2007;47:213–24.
14. Mehle ME, Kremer PS. Sinus CT scan findings in "sinus headache" migraineurs. Headache 2008;48:67–71.
15. Cady RK, Schreiber CP. Sinus headache: a clinical conundrum. Otolaryngol Clin North Am 2004;37:267–88.
16. Behin F, Lipton RB, Bigal M. Migraine and intranasal contact point headache: is there any connection? Curr Pain Headache Rep 2006;10:312–5.
17. Jackson A, Dial A. Sinus headache in an ENT setting. Presented at the American Academy of Neurology Annual Meeting. Miami, Florida, April 9–16, 2004.

18. Tan BK, Chandra RK, Pollak J, et al. Incidence and associated premorbid diagnoses of patients with chronic rhinosinusitis. J Allergy Clin Immunol 2013;131: 1350–60.
19. Hsueh WD, Conley DB, Kim H, et al. Identifying clinical symptoms for improving the symptomatic diagnosis of chronic sinusitis. Int Forum Allergy Rhinol 2013;3: 307–14.
20. Cady RK, Schreiber CP. Sinus problems as a cause of headache refractoriness and migraine chronification. Curr Pain Headache Rep 2009;13:319–25.
21. Ku M, Silverman B, Prifti N, et al. Prevalence of migraine headaches in patients with allergic rhinitis. Ann Allergy Asthma Immunol 2006;97:226–30.
22. Martin VT, Taylor F, Gebhardt B, et al. Allergy and immunotherapy: are they related to migraine headache? Headache 2011;51:8–20.
23. Anon JB, Jacobs MR, Poole MD, et al, Sinus and Allergy Health Partnership. Antimicrobial treatment guidelines for acute bacterial rhinosinusitis–2004. Otolaryngol Head Neck Surg 2004;130(1):S1–50.
24. Clifton NJ, Jones NS. Prevalence of facial pain in 100 consecutive patients with paranasal mucopurulent discharge at endoscopy. J Laryngol Otol 2007;121: 345–8.
25. Soler ZM, Mace J, Smith TL. Symptom-based presentation of chronic rhinosinusitis and symptom-specific outcomes after endoscopic sinus surgery. Am J Rhinol 2008;22:297–301.
26. Chester AC, Antisdel JL, Sindwani R. Symptom-specific outcomes of endoscopic sinus surgery: a systematic review. Otolaryngol Head Neck Surg 2009; 140:633–9.
27. Ahamed SH, Jones NS. What is Sluder's neuralgia? J Laryngol Otol 2003;117: 437–43.
28. Puig CM, Driscoll CL, Kern EB. Sluder's sphenopalatine ganglion neuralgia-treatment with 88% phenol. Am J Rhinol 1998;12:113–8.
29. Wolff HG. The nasal, paranasal, and aural structures as sources of headache and other pain. In: Headache and other head pain. New York: Oxford University Press; 1948. p. 532–60.
30. Abu-Bakra M, Jones NS. Does stimulation of nasal mucosa cause referred pain to the face? Clin Otolaryngol 2001;26:430–2.
31. Abu-Bakra M, Jones NS. The prevalence of nasal contact points in a population with facial pain and a control population. J Laryngol Otol 2001;115: 626–32.
32. Bieger-Farhan AK, Nichani J, Willat DJ. Nasal septal contact points: associated symptoms and sinus CT scan scoring. Clin Otolaryngol Allied Sci 2004;29: 165–8.
33. Mariotti LJ, Setliff RC, Ghaderi M, et al. Patient history and CT findings in predicting surgical outcomes for patients with rhinogenic headache. Ear Nose Throat J 2009;88:926–9.
34. Goldsmith AJ, Zahtz GD, Stegnjajic A, et al. Middle turbinate headache syndrome. Am J Rhinol 1993;7:17–23.
35. Badran HS. Role of surgery in isolated concha bullosa. Clin Med Insights Ear Nose Throat 2011;4:13–9.
36. Kunachak S. Middle turbinate lateralization: a simple treatment for rhinologic headache. Laryngoscope 2002;112:870–2.
37. Sanges G, Feleppa M, Gamerra M, et al. Fronto-turbinalis sinus expansion and headache. Curr Pain Headache Rep 2011;15(4):308–13. http://dx.doi.org/10.1007/s11916-011-0194-2.

38. Ramadan HH. Nonsurgical versus endoscopic sinonasal surgery for rhinologic headache. Am J Rhinol 1999;13:455–7.
39. Abu-Samra M, Gawad OA, Agha M. The outcomes for nasal contact point surgeries in patients with unsatisfactory response to chronic daily headache medications. Eur Arch Otorhinolaryngol 2011;268:1299–304.
40. Bektas D, Alioglu Z, Akyol N, et al. Surgical outcomes for rhinogenic contact point headaches. Med Princ Pract 2011;20:29–33.
41. Patel ZM, Kennedy DW, Setzen M, et al. "Sinus headache": rhinogenic headache or migraine? An evidence-based guide to diagnosis and treatment. Int Forum Allergy Rhinol 2013;3:221–30.
42. Harrison L, Jones NS. Intranasal contact points as a cause of facial pain or headache: a systematic review. Clin Otolaryngol 2013;38:8–22.
43. Guyuron B, Reed D, Kriegler JS, et al. A placebo-controlled surgical trial of the treatment of migraine headaches. Plast Reconstr Surg 2009;124:461–8.
44. Guyuron B, Kriegler JS, Davis J, et al. Five-year outcome of surgical treatment of migraine headaches. Plast Reconstr Surg 2011;127:603–8.
45. Lee M, Monson MA, Liu MT, et al. Positive botulinum toxin type A response is a prognosticator for migraine surgery success. Plast Reconstr Surg 2013;131: 751–7.
46. Yazici ZM, Cabalar M, Sayin I, et al. Rhinologic evaluation in patients with primary headache. J Craniofac Surg 2010;21:1688–91.
47. Novak VJ, Makek M. Pathogenesis and surgical treatment of migraine and neurovascular headaches with rhinogenic trigger. Head Neck 1992;14:467–72.
48. Sindwani R, Wright ED. Role of endoscopic septoplasty in the treatment of atypical facial pain. J Otolaryngol 2003;32:77–80.
49. Mokbel KM, Abd Elfattah AM, Kamal E. Nasal mucosal contact points with facial pain and/or headache: lidocaine can predict the result the result of localized endoscopic resection. Eur Arch Otorhinolaryngol 2010;267:1569–72.
50. Mohebbi A, Memari F, Mohebbi S. Endonasal endoscopic management of contact point headache and diagnostic criteria. Headache 2010;50:242–8.

Evaluation and Management of "Sinus Headache" in the Otolaryngology Practice

Zara M. Patel, MD[a,*], Michael Setzen, MD[b],
David M. Poetker, MD[c], John M. DelGaudio, MD[a]

KEYWORDS

- Headache • Sinus headache • Rhinogenic headache • Migraine • Cluster headache
- Tension headache • Trigeminal autonomic cephalalgias

KEY POINTS

- Patients will believe pain or pressure over the sinus region is originating from the sinuses until you can prove otherwise, either by endoscopy or CT scan.
- Correct diagnosis can only come after completing a full history and physical, including nasal endoscopy, using imaging if indicated, and having a working knowledge of common headache diagnostic criteria.
- The most common primary headache syndrome that is mistakenly diagnosed as "sinus headache" is migraine.
- Although a neurologist is the best physician to evaluate and formulate a treatment strategy in patients with primary headache syndromes, there are a few straightforward initial treatment options that an otolaryngologist should be familiar with to try and alleviate the patient's symptoms as soon as possible.

INTRODUCTION

According to a worldwide Nielsen survey performed in 2007, headache is the most common complaint that leads people around the world to seek medical care.[1] Otolaryngologists see a large proportion of these patients, as people expect that if they have pain or pressure in their head and neck, that a head and neck doctor likely knows how to diagnose and treat the problem. Outside of primary care doctors and emergency

Financial Disclosures: Z.M. Patel has no financial disclosures; M. Setzen, Speakers Bureau for TEVA and Meda; D.M. Poetker has no financial disclosures; J.M. DelGaudio has no financial disclosures.
[a] Department of Otolaryngology/Head and Neck Surgery, Emory University School of Medicine, Atlanta, GA, USA; [b] North Shore University Hospital, New York University School of Medicine, New York, NY, USA; [c] Division of Otolaryngology, Department of Surgery, Zablocki VAMC, Milwaukee, WI, USA
* Corresponding author. Department of Otolaryngology/H&N Surgery, 550 Peachtree Street Northeast, 11th Floor, Atlanta, GA.
E-mail address: zara.m.patel@emory.edu

room physicians, otolaryngologists, neurologists, and oral surgeons see the majority of these patients.

Patients with pain in or around their sinonasal region often blame the sinuses for this pain based on the logical rationale that if a structure lies directly below the surface of the face where the pain or pressure is located, it is likely caused by a problem with this structure. There are also those patients who mistakenly assume they have sinuses where the pain/pressure is located because they do not know what else would cause such a sensation. Some patients will point to their temple and say the pain is coming from "that sinus." Patients are not the only ones guilty of this assumption. Many erroneous referrals for "sinus headache" are sent to otolaryngologists by primary care doctors and emergency room physicians. Although the mantra, "common things are common," is generally a respectable guide for these physicians, distinguishing between multiple common disorders in this region has been a problem and is now the focus of cross-specialty efforts to educate whichever physicians may see these patients first.[2]

There is good reason for confusion and misdiagnosis, because symptoms seen in multiple primary headache disorders as well as common rhinologic disorders overlap extensively. Otolaryngologists are often guilty of assuming all headaches not attributable to an ear, nose, and throat (ENT) disorder must be migraine. This review discusses the most common diagnoses that can masquerade as "sinus headache" or "rhinogenic headache", including the trigeminal autonomic cephalalgias (TACs), which include cluster headache (CH) and paroxysmal hemicrania (PH), hemicrania continua (HC), trigeminal neuralgia (TN), and tension-type headache (TTH); temporomandibular joint dysfunction (TMD); giant cell arteritis (GCA), which is also known as temporal arteritis; medication overuse headache (MOH); and migraine. We will go through the diagnostic criteria for each and outline the evidence that will allow physicians to make better clinical diagnoses and point their patients toward better treatment options.

DIAGNOSTIC CRITERIA

First published in 1997 and then revised in 2003, a rhinosinusitis task force (RTF) established by the American Academy of Otolaryngology–Head and Neck Surgery designated criteria for the diagnosis of acute and chronic rhinosinusitis, which are set forth in **Tables 1–3**.[3–5] Facial pressure or pain must be combined with at least one other major factor to warrant a chronic sinusitis diagnosis; each is not enough on its own.

Table 1	
RTF definition of major and minor factors in the diagnosis of sinusitis in adults	
Major Factors	**Minor Factors**
Facial pain/pressure (must be associated with another major factor)	Headache
Facial congestion/fullness	Fever (must be associated with another major nasal symptom)
Nasal obstruction/blockage	Halitosis
Nasal discharge/drainage	Fatigue
Hyposmia/anosmia	Dental pain
Fever (in acute)	Cough Ear pain/pressure/fullness

From Lanza DC, Kennedy DW. Adult rhinosinusitis defined. Otolaryngol Head Neck Surg 1997;117(pt 2):S1–7; with permission.

Table 2
RTF definitions of acute and chronic sinusitis

Acute Sinusitis	Chronic Sinusitis
Duration 4 or less weeks	Duration 12 or more weeks
2 or More major factors OR	2 or More major factors OR
1 Major + 2 minor factors OR	1 Major + 2 minor factors OR
Nasal purulence on examination	Nasal purulence on examination

From Lanza DC, Kennedy DW. Adult rhinosinusitis defined. Otolaryngol Head Neck Surg 1997;117(pt 2):S1–7; with permission.

The International Headache Society (IHS) has diagnostic criteria for all headache syndromes, and the criteria for the headache disorders are in **Boxes 1–9** and **Table 4**.[5]

The current evidence available in the literature is scarce with regard to diagnostic studies directly comparing rhinogenic causes with temporomandibular joint dysfunction, tension type headache, medication overuse headache, giant cell arteritis, and trigeminal neuralgia. Simply knowing the different diagnostic criteria may be enough, however, in selecting these possible causes of headache and facial pain; these differences are reviewed. In contrast, there are some studies showing how frequently the trigeminal autonomic cephalalgias headache disorders are incorrectly diagnosed as sinus-related disorders and significant evidence that helps distinguish migraine from rhinogenic causes.

Importantly, the IHS notes that chronic sinusitis is "not validated as a cause of headache or facial pain unless relapsing into an acute stage". Also of interest is that mucosal contact point headache has a place within the appendix A11.5.1 of the IHS classification system, as a cause of headache "for which evidence is limited". We will lay out that evidence as well, later in this review.

ESTABLISHING DIAGNOSIS

The key to finding the right diagnosis in each individual presenting with "sinus headache" is to perform a stepwise, comprehensive evaluation of the patient, including an extensive history, thorough head and neck examination (including neurologic examination), nasal endoscopy, CT scan, and application of IHS criteria.

It is noted clearly in the neurologic literature that the history is the most important part of the patient appointment, and 99% of a physician's time should be spent on

Table 3
2003 RTF revised criteria to also include 1 of the following for the diagnosis of chronic sinusitis

Discolored nasal drainage from the nasal passages, nasal polyps, or polypoid swelling as identified on physical examination with anterior rhinoscopy after decongestion or nasal endoscopy

Edema or erythema of the middle meatus or ethmoid bulla on nasal endoscopy

Generalized or localized erythema, edema, or granulation tissue (if the middle meatus or ethmoid bulla is not involved, radiologic imaging is required to confirm a diagnosis)

CT scanning demonstrating isolated or diffuse mucosal thickening, bone changes, or air-fluid levels OR

Plain sinus radiography revealing air-fluid levels or greater than 5 mm of opacification of 1 or more sinuses

From Benninger MS, Ferguson BJ, Hadley JA, et al. Adult chronic rhinosinusitis: definitions, diagnosis, epidemiology, and pathophysiology. Otolaryngol Head Neck Surg 2003;129:S1–32; with permission.

Box 1
IHS diagnostic criteria for headache attributed to rhinosinusitis

1. Frontal headache accompanied by pain in 1 or more regions of the face, ears, or teeth and fulfilling criteria 3 and 4

2. Clinical, nasal endoscopic, CT and/or MRI, and/or laboratory evidence of acute or acute-on-chronic rhinosinusitis[a]

3. Headache and facial pain develop simultaneously with onset or acute exacerbation of rhinosinusitis

4. Headache and/or facial pain resolve within 7 days after remission or successful treatment of acute or acute-on-chronic rhinosinusitis

   [a] Clinical evidence may include purulence in the nasal cavity, nasal obstruction, hyposmia, anosmia, and/or fever.
   From Cady RJ, Dodick DW, Levine HL, et al. Sinus headache: a neurology, otolaryngology, allergy and primary care consensus on diagnosis and treatment. Mayo Clin Proc 2005;80(7):908–16; with permission.

---

gaining a complete history.[6,7] However, when a patient arrives in an otolaryngologist's office, the onus is on that physician to not only diagnose the true cause of pain and pressure to the best of his/her ability but also to rule out any ENT-related issues that could cause those symptoms. Thus, nasal endoscopy (preferably that patients can also witness on a monitor) becomes paramount to showing what may or may not be going on inside the nasal cavity and why this may or may not be the cause of the headache, especially if contact points can be demonstrated, or that there is simply a normal examination.

To separate rhinogenic headache from temporomandibular joint dysfunction is simple based on signs and symptoms. The Research Diagnostic Criteria for Temporomandibular Disorders (RDC/TMD) are widely used and these criteria are published online. The protocol itself is an 89-page document and is not republished in this

---

Box 2
IHS diagnostic criteria for headache attributed to temporomandibular joint dysfunction

A. Recurrent pain in 1 or more regions of the head and/or face, fulfilling criteria C and D

B. Radiograph, MRI, or bone scintigraphy demonstrates temporomandibular joint (TMD) disorder

C. Evidence that pain can be attributed to the TMD disorder, based on at least 1 of the following:

   1. Pain is precipitated by jaw movements and/or chewing of hard or tough food

   2. Reduced range of or irregular jaw opening

   3. Noise from 1 or both TMDs during jaw movements

   4. Tenderness of the joint capsule(s) of 1 or both TMDs

D. Headache resolves within 3 months and does not recur after successful treatment of the TMD disorder

From Headache Classification Subcommittee of the International Headache Society. The international classification of headache disorders: 2nd edition. Cephalalgia 2004;24(Suppl 1):9–160; with permission.

article, but key points are summarized. TMD is separated into 2 axes. Axis I allows the classification of TMD in 3 subtypes: muscular (also known as myofascial), intra-articular, and arthritic. Axis II assesses the severity of the pain caused by the TMD.[8] Articular TMD is the easiest to differentiate from rhinogenic problems due to the classic clicking and popping associated with jaw opening and crepitus that can usually be palpated over the joint. Even when the pain of this joint radiates forward across the cheek and upward toward the temple, these obvious clues allow a physician to hone in on this joint as the source of pain. The myofascial type is more difficult to differentiate, because it often is simply pain or pressure originating in the muscles of mastication as they strain to compensate for misalignment or labor under jaw clenching or other more subtle issues, and this can be harder to explain to patients when there are no classic joint-related symptoms. Either way, using the extensive criteria in the RDC/TMD allows a practitioner to diagnose this problem. History of jaw clenching or bruxism at night, signs of flattened cuspid ridges from grinding, classic pain with yawning, excessive talking, chewing and palpation over the joint with jaw opening and closing, and decreased range of motion are all significant findings that increase the likelihood of this diagnosis.[9]

Tension type headache is the most prevalent headache type, with up to 78% of the world's population experiencing it at least once.[10] However, not many experience them with enough frequency and severity, to bring them to a doctor's attention. It is generally described as a bandlike, squeezing headache around the frontal or temporal region, which can extend all the way around to include parietal and occipital regions as well. Due to the overlap in location of the frontal sinuses, it can be mistaken for frontal sinus disease. It can also be confused with TMD when the pain is in the temporal region and due to multiple overlapping symptoms can also be confused with migraine. Nasal endoscopy, physical examination, and CT scan if necessary to confirm or rule out pathologies in this region can help distinguish TTH from the other causes of headache.

Box 3
IHS diagnostic criteria for tension type headache

A. Headache lasting from 30 minutes to 7 days (or even more persistent if diagnosing chronic TTH)

B. Headache has at least 2 of the following characteristics:

   1. Bilateral location

   2. Pressing/tightening (nonpulsating) quality

   3. Mild or moderate intensity

   4. Not aggravated by routine physical activity, such as walking or climbing stairs

C. Both of the following:

   1. No nausea or vomiting (anorexia may occur)

   2. No more than one of phonophobia or photophobia

D. Not attributed to another disorder

From Headache Classification Subcommittee of the International Headache Society. The international classification of headache disorders: 2nd edition. Cephalalgia 2004;24(Suppl 1):9–160; with permission.

Box 4
IHS diagnostic criteria for classic trigeminal neuralgia

A. Paroxsysmal attacks of pain lasting from a fraction of a second to 2 minutes, affecting 1 or more divisions of the trigeminal nerve and fulfilling criteria B and C

B. Pain has at least 1 of the following characteristics:

1. Intense, sharp, superficial, or stabbing

2. Precipitated from trigger areas or trigger factors

C. Attacks are stereotyped in the individual patient

D. There is no clinically evident neurologic deficit

E. Not attributed to another disorder

From Headache Classification Subcommittee of the International Headache Society. The international classification of headache disorders: 2nd edition. Cephalalgia 2004;24(Suppl 1):9–160; with permission.

Another diagnosis that can become apparent simply through close attention to history is Trigeminal Neuralgia (TN). TN is a unilateral disorder characterized by brief, sudden electric shock–like pain that is limited to the distribution of the trigeminal nerve and is abrupt in onset and termination. The pain can be spontaneous or it can be elicited by a trigger factor, such as washing the face or brushing the teeth. Naturally when this occurs, patients think the pain is related to the structure they have just touched and what is located beneath the surface of the skin, which is often a sinus cavity, especially when V2 is the branch involved.[5] Sinus disease has never been associated with this type of sharp, stabbing pain, however, and although a convincing diagnosis can be made on history alone, nasal endoscopy with or without CT scan is performed simply to demonstrate this to the patient. The 2 variants of TN are "classic" and "symptomatic". The symptomatic type is simply when the cranial nerve symptom is actually a sign of another pathology. The classic type is almost always unilateral, except in the rare instance of a central cause, such as multiple sclerosis. As posterior fossa exploration and MRI have become more common, the literature suggests that many, if not all, of these patients have compression of the trigeminal nerve root by aberrant vessels.

Giant Cell Arteritis (GCA) is another commonly unilateral headache syndrome, although it can be bilateral. Pain on chewing from jaw claudication is a common presenting symptom and this often leads to misdiagnosis as TMD. Some of these patients end up in a rhinologist's office after a clean bill of health from a local dentist, with the suggestion that they have sinusitis. Epidemiology can be helpful in this situation, with GCA affecting women 3 times more often than men with a mean age of onset of 70 years. If there is a huge, swollen, painful temporal artery pulsating on examination, the diagnosis may be simple. The presentation may not always be clear, however, and elevated erythrocyte sedimentation rate (ESR) ESR or C-reactive protein (CRP) may prompt the physician to perform a temporal artery biopsy. Due to the variable location of the arteritis within the vessel, false-negative rate results can be high, but the biopsy likely is more helpful if it is directed by a duplex study to regions that show a halo sign, demonstrating wall thickening.[11]

Box 5
IHS diagnostic criteria for giant cell arteritis

A. Any new persisting headache fulfilling criteria C and D

B. At least 1 of the following:

1. Swollen tender scalp artery with elevated ESR or CRP

2. Temporal artery biopsy demonstrating GCA

C. Headache develops in close temporal relation to other symptoms and signs of GCA (these may include jaw claudication, polymyalgia rheumatica, recent repeated attacks of amaurosis fugax)[a]

D. Headache resolves within 3 days of high-dose steroid treatment

[a] Signs and symptoms may be so variable that any recent persisting HA in a patient over 60 years old should suggest this diagnosis. There is a major risk of blindness that is preventable by immediate steroid treatment and the time interval between visual loss in one eye and in the other is usually less than a week.

From Headache Classification Subcommittee of the International Headache Society. The international classification of headache disorders: 2nd edition. Cephalalgia 2004;24(Suppl 1):9–160; with permission.

Medication Overuse headache (MOH) is a very complex diagnosis. This is due to multiple confounding symptoms and signs, the fact that patients likely have a primary headache disorder that will eventually be diagnosed once the medication is stopped, and also due to extreme patient resistance to this diagnosis. Again, the key to full understanding is the history. If a physician takes the time to listen to patients and validates their headache and pain, the reception to a diagnosis of MOH is different than when patients feel they were not heard. Also, it is only a trusting patient who divulges to a doctor the extent of medication overuse. Without building a bond of mutual respect and understanding, it is doubtful that physicians will have the chance to make a correct diagnosis in these patients. Clinical features depend on the substance of overuse. For example, patients overusing ergot or analgesics suffer from a tension-like daily headache, but those patients who overuse triptans complain of migraine-like daily headache or increase in frequency of migraines.[12] When these types of headaches are easily confused with "sinus headache", otolaryngologists are bound to see many patients in their office who are suffering from this problem.

Box 6
IHS diagnostic criteria for medication overuse headache

A. Headache present on ≥15 days/month fulfilling criteria C and D

B. Regular overuse for ≥3 months of 1 or more drugs that can be taken for acute and/or symptomatic treatment of headache

C. Headache has developed or markedly worsened during medication overuse

D. Headache resolves or reverts to its previous pattern within 2 months of discontinuation of overused medication

From Headache Classification Subcommittee of the International Headache Society. The international classification of headache disorders: 2nd edition. Cephalalgia 2004;24(Suppl 1):9–160; with permission.

Box 7
IHS diagnostic criteria for cluster headache

A. At least 5 attacks fulfilling criteria B–D

B. Severe or very severe unilateral orbital, supraorbital, and/or temporal pain lasting 15–180 minutes if untreated

C. Headache is accompanied by at least 1 of the following:

    1. Ipsilateral conjunctival injection and/or lacrimation

    2. Ipsilateral nasal congestion and/or rhinorrhea

    3. Ipsilateral eyelid edema

    4. Ipsilateral forehead and facial sweating

    5. Ipsilateral miosis and/or ptosis

    6. A sense of restlessness or agitation

D. Attacks have a frequency from 1 every other day to 8 per day

E. Not attributed to another disorder

From Headache Classification Subcommittee of the International Headache Society. The international classification of headache disorders: 2nd edition. Cephalalgia 2004;24(Suppl 1):9–160; with permission.

The trigeminal autonomic cephalalgia headache disorders and Hemicrania Continua (HC) are frequently misdiagnosed as having a rhinogenic source due to the ipsilateral autonomic symptoms that are part of these diagnoses, such as nasal congestion, rhinorrhea, eyelid edema, ptosis or miosis, and conjunctival injection

Box 8
IHS diagnostic criteria for paroxysmal hemicrania

A. At least 20 attacks fulfilling criteria B–D

B. Attacks of severe unilateral orbital, supraorbital, or temporal pain lasting 2–30 minutes

C. Headache is accompanied by at least 1 of the following:

    1. Ipsilateral conjunctival injection and/or lacrimation

    2. Ipsilateral nasal congestion and/or rhinorrhea

    3. Ipsilateral eyelid edema

    4. Ipsilateral forehead or facial sweating

    5. Ipsilateral miosis and/or ptosis

D. Attacks have a frequency above 5 per day for more than half the time, although periods with lower frequency may occur

E. Attacks are prevented completely by therapeutic doses of indomethacin (in order to rule out incomplete response) and should be used in a dose of $\geq$150 mg qd orally or rectally, or $\geq$100 mg IV, but for maintenance, smaller doses are often sufficient

F. Not attributed to another disorder

From Headache Classification Subcommittee of the International Headache Society. The international classification of headache disorders: 2nd edition. Cephalalgia 2004;24(Suppl 1):9–160; with permission.

Box 9
IHS diagnostic criteria for hemicrania continua

A. Headache for >3 months fulfilling criteria B–D

B. All of the following characteristics:

   1. Unilateral pain without side shift

   2. Daily and continuous without pain-free periods

   3. Moderate intensity but with exacerbations of severe pain

C. At least 1 of the following autonomic features occurs during exacerbations and ipsilateral to the side of the pain:

   1. Conjunctival injection and/or lacrimation

   2. Nasal congestion and/or rhinorrhea

   3. Ptosis and/or miosis

D. Complete response to therapeutic doses of indomethacin

E. Not attributed to another disorder

From Headache Classification Subcommittee of the International Headache Society. The international classification of headache disorders: 2nd edition. Cephalalgia 2004;24(Suppl 1):9–160; with permission.

---

and lacrimation. A review was performed in 2013 looking at errors in diagnosis or therapy for these headache syndromes, and 22 articles were found relevant and met the authors' inclusion criteria.[13] They found that migraine with and without aura, TN, sinus infection, dental pain, and temporomandibular dysfunction were the disorders most frequently overdiagnosed in spite of the clear-cut criteria the IHS has published for diagnosing trigeminal autonomic cephalalgias. **Tables 5–7** summarize the articles

---

Table 4
IHS diagnostic criteria for migraine

Migraine with Aura	Migraine Without Aura
1. At least 2 attacks fulfilling criteria 2–4 if aura is present	1. At least 5 attacks fulfilling criteria 2–4 when aura is not present
2. Headache lasts 4–72 h	2. Headache lasts 4–72 h
3. Headache that has 2 of the following: unilateral, pulsating quality, moderate or severe pain intensity, aggravated by or causing avoidance of routine physical activity	3. Headache that has 2 of the following: unilateral, pulsating quality, moderate or severe pain intensity, aggravated by or causing avoidance of routine physical activity
4. One of the following occurs during the headache: nausea, vomiting, photophobia, phonophobia	4. One of the following occurs during the headache: nausea, vomiting, photophobia, phonophobia
5. Headache cannot be attributed to another disorder	5. Headache cannot be attributed to another disorder

From Kari E, DelGaudio JM. Treatment of sinus headache as migraine: the diagnostic utility of triptans. Laryngoscope 2008;118:2235–9; with permission.

Table 5
Summary of studies (with >10 patients) showing erroneous diagnosis in cluster headache

Study/Year	Number of Subjects	Misdiagnoses	Treatments Performed Prior to Obtaining Correct Diagnosis of CH
Bittar and Graff-Radford,[14] 1992	33	Not reported	42% of Patients received inappropriate dental treatment, which was often irreversible, almost all patients received different medications (NSAIDs, opiates, AEDs, TCAs).
Klapper et al,[15] 2000	693	3.9 (Average number of incorrect diagnoses before CH) NOS	5% Had surgery (mostly sinus or deviated septum surgery); other patients were prescribed multiple sinus medications.
van Vliet et al,[16] 2003	1163	Sinusitis (21%), migraine (17%), dental-related pain (11%)	Tooth extraction (16%) and ENT operation (12%).
Bahra and Goadsby,[17] 2004	230	Not reported	52% of Patients who had been seen by a dentist or ENT surgeon had an invasive procedure.
Jensen et al,[18] 2007	85	Not reported	Surgical treatment was received by 58% (49/85) of the cluster patients.
Van Alboom et al,[19] 2009	85	Migraine (45%), sinusitis (23%), tooth problems (23%), TTH (16%), TN (16%), ophthalmologic (10%), neck (7%), sinonasal (5%)	31% of Patients had invasive therapy prior to CH diagnosis, including dental procedures (21%) and sinus surgery (10%).

Data from Refs.[14–19]

reviewed and the findings therein, demonstrating a troublesome tableau of otolaryngologists, oral surgeons, and dentists performing unindicated procedures on these patients before they were finally correctly diagnosed.[14–28]

Migraine headache is a diagnosis that at times is clear and obvious but many other times is a difficult one, especially when dealing with migraine without aura. Of all the different headache syndromes, there exists the highest level of evidence for the misdiagnosis of migraine as "sinus headache". In contrast to the many case reports and small case series in the literature about the other headache syndromes diagnosed as "sinus headache" or headache with rhinogenic cause, there are multiple strong prospective cohort studies demonstrating the misdiagnosis of migraine as "sinus headache". A summary of these studies is in **Table 8**. The literature confirms that when a patient presents with a "sinus headache" diagnosis but has clear sinuses on endoscopy and CT scan, the most likely correct diagnosis is migraine.[29–34]

Table 6
Summary of studies showing erroneous diagnosis in paroxysmal hemicrania

Study/Year	Number of Subjects	Misdiagnoses	Treatments Performed Prior to Obtaining Correct Diagnosis of PH
Delcanho and Graff-Redford,[20] 1993	2	Case 1: dental pain, migraine Case 2: TN, TMD	Case 1: Randomized clinical trial, migraine prophylactic medications Case 2: phenytoin 100 mg tid
Moncada and Graff-Redford,[21] 1995	1	TMD	Complete mouth reconstruction, then recommendation having condyloplasty
Benoliel and Sharav,[22] 1998	7	Pain of dental origin, TMD, CH	1 Tooth extraction, 1 root canal, 1 received antibiotics
Sarlani et al,[23] 2003	1	TN and sinusitis	Maxillary sinus surgery, carbamazapine, prednisone, paracetomol
Alonso and Nixdorf,[24] 2006	1	TMD	Splint therapy and bite adjustments

Data from Refs.[20–24]

Table 7
Summary of studies showing erroneous diagnosis in hemicrania continua

Study/Year	Number of Subjects	Misdiagnoses	Treatments Performed Prior to Obtaining Correct Diagnosis of HC
Benoliel et al,[25] 2002	1	Dental pain, migraine, cervicogenic headache (CEH)	Dental treatment (Not otherwise specified), intensive physiotherapy, paracetamol, propranolol, diazepam, ergotamine combination, diclofenac sodium.
Alonso and Nixdorf,[24] 2006	1	Dental pain, CEH	Dental extraction, cervical adjustment, multiple chronic pain medications.
Taub et al,[26] 2008	2	TMD, dental pain, CH, migraine	Topiramate, nortriptyline, melatonin, verapamil, gabapentin.
Rossi et al,[27] 2009	25	Migraine (52%), CH (28%), sinus headache (20%), dental pain (20%), atypical facial pain (16%), stress headache (16%), CEH (8%)	NSAIDs (92%), triptans (32%), antidepressants (32%), and antiepileptics (24%). 36% Received invasive treatments.
Prakash et al,[28] 2010	4	Atypical facial pain, atypical odontalgia, sinusitis, caries, pulpitis, psychiatric disorder, chronic migraine	All the patients had dental extractions (6 in one patient), some had sinus surgery, root canal treatment.

Data from Refs.[24–28]

Table 8
Summary of diagnosis of "sinus headache" studies pointing to migraine

Study/Year	Study Design	Level of Evidence	Number of Subjects	Diagnostic Criteria	Conclusions
Barbanti et al,[29] 2002	Prospective cohort	2b	177	IHS criteria	Almost half of migraine patients exhibit unilateral cranial autonomic symptoms.
Perry et al,[30] 2004	Prospective cohort	2b	36	IHS criteria	Majority of patients with primary headache complaint in a tertiary rhinology practice have migraine.
Schreiber et al,[31] 2004	Prospective cohort	2b	2991	IHS criteria	Migraine with or without aura is diagnosis of "sinus headache" patient majority of the time.
Eross et al,[32] 2004	Prospective cohort	1b	100	IHS criteria	Majority of patients with "sinus headache" diagnosed with migraine. Most common reason for prior misdiagnosis was triggers, provocation, and location.
Mehle and Kremer,[33] 2008	Prospective cohort	2b	35	IHS criteria	Majority of patients with "sinus headache" diagnosed with migraine. Positive migraine history does not obviate thorough ENT work-up because some of these patients have positive sinus CT scans.
Foroughipour et al,[34] 2011	Prospective cohort	2b	58	IHS criteria	Majority of patients with "sinus headache" have migraine.

Data from Refs.[29–34]

RECOMMENDING TREATMENT

If a diagnostician is skilled enough to wade through the multiple overlapping symptoms and signs in patients with "sinus headache" and is able to come to a correct diagnosis, what can then be done to treat these patients?

If patients truly are found to have acute or chronic sinusitis as a cause of the headache, then treatment should be initiated immediately to address this issue. There are a plethora of recommendations in the treatment of rhinosinusitis, and an exhaustive review of these is beyond the scope of this review. Readers are referred to the recent European Position Paper on Rhinosinusitis and Nasal Polyps 2012 for a comprehensive review of these subjects.[35]

For headache syndromes that are a neurologist's specialty, otolaryngologists are cautioned to refer patients to neurology colleagues for a comprehensive evaluation and treatment strategy. There are a few of these disorders, however, where getting patients started in the right direction is straightforward and will help to alleviate their symptoms until a neurology appointment is obtained.

For example, there are few treatments as straightforward as that for paroxysmal hemicrania (PH) and Hemicrania Continua (HC). Response to indomethacin even makes it into the diagnostic criteria for these disorders, and the complete alleviation of headache results in a grateful patient. As noted in **Box 8**, in order to rule out incomplete response, indomethacin should be used in a dose of greater than or equal to 150 mg per day orally or rectally or greater than or equal to 100 mg intravenous (IV), but for maintenance, smaller doses are often sufficient.[5]

For Cluster Headache (CH), there is a lot of research ongoing for those patients who do not respond to first-line therapy, but in general, for acute treatment of CH attacks, oxygen (100%), with a flow of at least 7 L/min over 15 minutes and sumatriptan (6 mg subcutaneous) are the drugs of first choice. Prophylaxis of CH should be performed with verapamil at a daily dose of at least 240 mg (with the maximum dose depending on efficacy and/or tolerability). Although the level of evidence is lower, steroids are clearly effective in cluster headache. Therefore, the use of at least 100 mg methylprednisolone (or equivalent corticosteroid) given orally or up to 500 mg IV per day over 5 days (then tapering down) is also recommended, if no contraindication exists. Methysergide, lithium, and topiramate have been suggested as alternative treatments. Surgical procedures, targeting the sphenopalatine ganglion with methods such as injection of anesthetic or radiofrequency ablation, are a new area of interest and require further study to assess true efficacy.[36]

The treatment of tension type headache is complex and involves the use of over-the-counter medications, such as acetaminophen, aspirin, and nonsteroidal anti-inflammatory drugs (NSAIDs), as well as stronger muscle relaxants, antidepressants, such as the tricyclic antidepressants (TCAs), and therapy such as cognitive behavioral counseling and biofeedback. All have been used to some efficacy in this headache disorder.[10]

As most otolaryngologists know, the treatment of temporomandibular joint dysfunction starts out conservatively and then can range to invasive procedures. A review looking at the range of therapies concluded that dentists and surgeons treating these patients have an ethical obligation to start with conservative, noninvasive, nonirreversible therapies, such as education, behavior avoidance, oral appliances, and splints, before moving to occlusion-changing interventions and joint surgery.[37]

There is a wide range of medical and surgical treatments available for trigeminal neuralgia, and due to the controversy surrounding etiology and pathophysiology, there probably will be continuous development of treatment until this disorder is better understood. The current preferred medical treatment of trigeminal neuralgia consists of anticonvulsant drugs, muscle relaxants, and neuroleptic agents. Large-scale, placebo-controlled clinical trials are scarce. For patients refractory to medical therapy, Gasserian ganglion percutaneous techniques, Gamma-knife surgery, and microvascular decompression are the most promising invasive treatment options.[38]

Giant Cell Arteritis (GCA), or temporal arteritis, is a dangerous diagnosis if not treated promptly and correctly and can lead to blindness or even aortic aneurysm if left unchecked. The treatment of choice is steroids, but there is a lack of consensus as to the appropriate starting dose; 40–60 mg is the usual starting dose, although some ophthalmologists have voiced concern at starting at a dose lower than 60 mg due to possible visual compromise at lower doses. This higher dose (that patients will have to stay at, in some cases, for an extended period of time) should be weighed against the risks of high-dose steroids. The length of treatment also lacks consensus but it seems that most patients can be weaned completely off steroid therapy within 2 years of diagnosis.[11]

Medication Overuse Headache (MOH) has only one possible treatment and that is complete withdrawal of medication. Therapy must consist of patient education, medication withdrawal including rescue medication, preventive treatment, and a multimodal approach including psychological support if necessary. The choice between inpatient and outpatient withdrawal model has not been conclusively determined, but most experts recommend inpatient treatment if the overused medications include barbiturates, codeine, or tranquilizers, for patients who failed to withdraw as outpatients on other medications, or for those who have a high depression score.[39]

The treatment of migraine is, at least at the outset, straightforward, and involves the use of triptans for abortive therapy. There are other medications, such as sodium valproate, that can then be used for preventive therapy, but, again, preventive therapy strategies are best managed by a trained neurologist. Of note, there are several studies using migraine therapies to empirically diagnose migraine in patients presenting with "sinus headache".[2,40–42] A summary of these studies is in **Table 9**. These findings suggest that if a rhinologist sees a patient with "sinus headache", the sinuses are clear on endoscopy and CT scan, and the symptoms and signs are not definitively pointing toward one of the other headache etiologies listed above, a trial of an abortive triptan medication is the next best step while the patient is awaiting an appointment with neurology.

One last controversial but possible cause of actual rhinogenic headache is the "contact point" headache. The authors do not believe this subset is a significant contributor to a large percentage of these patients. However, although no high-level evidence exists either way, there have been enough lower-level studies suggesting some benefit; thus, the evidence is discussed. Often in these studies, complications from surgery are not reported and follow-up is lacking. In spite of these shortcomings, however, there seems to be a select patient population who may possibly benefit from directed nasal surgery. They are those who have contact points, have failed medical therapy directed at primary headache diagnoses by a neurologist, have otherwise normal endoscopy and CT scan, and have improvement in headache symptoms after local application of an anesthetic to the contact point. Even in this patient population, an otolaryngologist should hold a lengthy discussion with respect to risks, benefits, and alternatives, with emphasis on the fact that surgery may not alleviate the facial pain and/or headache.[43–46] A summary of these studies is in **Table 10**.

Table 9
Summary of treatment of "sinus headache" as migraine studies

Study/Year	Study Design	Level of Evidence	Number of Subjects	Study Groups	Protocol	Primary Endpoint	Conclusion
Cady et al,[2] 2005	Prospective cohort	2b	47	Sumatriptan	2 doses 50 mg	Reduction of moderate to severe headaches to mild or no pain	Majority of patients with "sinus headche" are effectively treated with migraine-directed therapy.
Kari and DelGaudio,[40] 2008	Prospective cohort	2b	54	Elatriptan or other migraine-directed therapy	40 mg For every headache over 1–3 mo	50% Reduction in frequency and severity of headaches	Large majority of patients with "sinus headache" are effectively treated with migraine-directed therapy, and this treatment may aid in diagnosis.
Dadgarnia et al,[41] 2010	Prospective cohort	2b	104	Sodium valproate	Daily over 6 mo	Improvement based on pain visual analog scale	Migraine-directed therapy is effective in majority of "sinus headache" patients.
Ishkanian et al,[42] 2007	Randomized clinical trial	1b	216	Sumatriptan	1 dose 50 mg	Reduction to no or mild pain on 4-point pain scale	Sumatriptan is effective in treating patients with "sinus headache".

Data from Refs.[2,40–42]

Table 10
Summary of treatment of mucosal contact points in patients with "sinus headache"

Study/Year	Study Design	Level of Evidence	Number of Subjects	Study Groups	Surgical Protocol	Primary Endpoint	Conclusion
Novak and Makek,[43] 1992	Prospective cohort	4	299	Frequent or pharmacologically resistant migraine	None specified	Subjective improvement	Surgery is a successful approach to patients with headache and mucosal contact points.
Tosun et al,[44] 2000	Prospective cohort	4	30	Contact point with no other cause of headache	Directed to only address contact points	Subjective improvement	Surgery is a successful approach to patients with headache from no other cause and mucosal contact points.
Welge-Luessen et al,[45] 2003	Prospective cohort	4	20	Refractory migraine or CH with contact points	None specified	Subjective improvement	Surgery is a successful approach to patients with headache and mucosal contact points.
Yazici et al,[46] 2010	Prospective cohort	4	73	Migraine or TTN with contact points	None specfied	Improvement on pain visual analog scale	Some patients with primary headache and contact points benefit from nasal surgery.

Data from Refs.[43–46]

A CAVEAT

A weak point remains, and a large one at that, in the effort to completely categorize patients presenting with "sinus headache". This is the group of patients who may, in fact, have minimal or mild mucosal changes in their sinuses. As is well known, these can be incidental findings and likely do not correlate to any of the headache symptoms of which they are complaining. It remains difficult, however, to convince patients of this in the face of a positive radiology report and multiple surgeons willing to operate on this insignificant disease. There remains a complete dearth of literature looking specifically at this subset of patients with self- or physician-diagnosed "sinus headache" and mild mucosal changes on CT. This must be accepted as an inherent weakness of this overall review; further study is necessary in this patient population.

SUMMARY

Patients will continue to present to the otolaryngologist's office with headache as their primary complaint. If an otolaryngologist performs a directed history and comprehensive head and neck examination including nasal endoscopy, obtains imaging as necessary, and keeps at the ready the criteria for diagnosing the various headache disorders that may disguise themselves as sinonasal complaints, the correct diagnosis and treatment plan can be implemented. In addition, the patient population treated will be better off and extremely grateful for someone finally pointing them in a direction to obtain the relief they truly need.

REFERENCES

1. Available at: nz.nielsen.com/news/OTC_Aug07.shtml. Accessed January 6, 2013.
2. Cady RJ, Dodick DW, Levine HL, et al. Sinus headache: a neurology, otolaryngology, allergy and primary care consensus on diagnosis and treatment. Mayo Clin Proc 2005;80(7):908–16.
3. Lanza DC, Kennedy DW. Adult rhinosinusitis defined. Otolaryngol Head Neck Surg 1997;117:S1–7.
4. Benninger MS, Ferguson BJ, Hadley JA, et al. Adult chronic rhinosinusitis: definitions, diagnosis, epidemiology, and pathophysiology. Otolaryngol Head Neck Surg 2003;129:S1–32.
5. Headache Classification Subcommittee of the International Headache Society. The international classification of headache disorders: 2nd edition. Cephalalgia 2004;24(Suppl 1):9–160.
6. Peatfield R. Headache and facial pain. Medicine 2008;36(10):526–30.
7. Bendtsen L, Jensen R. Tension-type headache. Neurol Clin 2009;27(2):525–35.
8. Dworkin SF, LeResche L. Research diagnostic criteria for temporomandibular disorders: review, criteria, examinations and specification, critique. J Craniomandib Disord 1992;6:310–54.
9. Lupoli TA, Lockey RF. Temporomandibular dysfunction: an often overlooked cause of chronic headache. Ann Allergy Asthma Immunol 2007;99:314–8.
10. Freitag F. Managing and treating tension type headache. Med Clin North Am 2013;97:281–92.
11. Waldman CW, Waldman SD, Waldman RA. Giant cell arteritis. Med Clin North Am 2013;97:329–35.
12. Katsarava Z, Obermann M. Medication overuse headache. Curr Opin Neurol 2013;26:276–81.

13. Viana M, Tassorelli C, Allena M, et al. Diagnostic and therapeutic errors in trigeminal autonomic cephalalgias and hemicrania continua: a systematic review. J Headache Pain 2013;14:14.

14. Bittar G, Graff-Radford SB. A retrospective study of patients with cluster headaches. Oral Surg Oral Med Oral Pathol 1992;14(5):519–25.

15. Klapper JA, Klapper A, Voss T. The misdiagnosis of cluster headache: a non-clinic, population-based, internet survey. Headache 2000;14(9):730–5.

16. van Vliet JA, Eekers PJ, Haan J, et al. Features involved in the diagnostic delay of cluster headache. J Neurol Neurosurg Psychiatry 2003;14(8):1123–5.

17. Bahra A, Goadsby PJ. Diagnostic delays and mis-management in cluster headache. Acta Neurol Scand 2004;14(3):175–9.

18. Jensen RM, Lyngberg A, Jensen RH. Burden of cluster headache. Cephalalgia 2007;14(6):535–41.

19. Van Alboom E, Louis P, Van Zandijcke M, et al. Diagnostic and therapeutic trajectory of cluster headache patients in Flanders. Acta Neurol Belg 2009;14(1):10–7.

20. Delcanho RE, Graff-Radford SB. Chronic paroxysmal hemicrania presenting as toothache. J Orofac Pain 1993;14(3):300–6.

21. Moncada E, Graff-Radford SB. Benign indomethacin-responsive headaches presenting in the orofacial region: eight case reports. J Orofac Pain 1995;14(3):276–84.

22. Benoliel R, Sharav Y. Paroxysmal hemicrania. Case studies and review of the literature. Oral Surg Oral Med Oral Pathol Oral Radiol Endod 1998;14(3):285–92.

23. Sarlani E, Schwartz AH, Greenspan JD, et al. Chronic paroxysmal hemicrania: a case report and review of the literature. J Orofac Pain 2003;14(1):74–8.

24. Alonso AA, Nixdorf DR. Case series of four different headache types presenting as tooth pain. J Endod 2006;14(11):1110–3.

25. Benoliel R, Robinson S, Eliav E, et al. Hemicrania continua. J Orofac Pain 2002; 16(4):317–25.

26. Taub D, Stiles A, Tucke AG. Hemicrania continua presenting as temporomandibular joint pain. Oral Surg Oral Med Oral Pathol Oral Radiol Endod 2008;14(2): e35–7.

27. Rossi P, Faroni J, Tassorelli C, et al. Diagnostic delay and suboptimal management in a referral population with hemicrania continua. Headache 2009;14(2):227–34.

28. Prakash S, Shah ND, Chavda BV. Unnecessary extractions in patients with hemicrania continua: case reports and implication for dentistry. J Orofac Pain 2010; 14(4):408–11.

29. Barbanti P, Fabbrini G, Pesare M, et al. Unilateral cranial autonomic symptoms in migraine. Cephalalgia 2002;22:256–9.

30. Perry BF, Login IS, Kountakis SE. Nonrhinologic headache in a tertiary rhinology practice. Otolaryngol Head Neck Surg 2004;130:449–52.

31. Schreiber CP, Hutchinson S, Webster CJ, et al. Prevalence of migraine among patients with history of self-reported or physician-diagnosed "sinus" headache. Arch Inten Med 2004;164:1769–72.

32. Eross EJ, Dodick DW, Eross MD. The sinus, allergy and migraine study (SAMS). Headache 2007;47:213–24.

33. Mehle ME, Kremer PS. Sinus CT scan findings in "sinus headache" migraineurs. Headache 2008;48:67–71.

34. Foroughipour M, Sharifian SM, Shoeibi A, et al. Causes of sinus headache in patients with a primary diagnosis of sinus headache. Eur Arch Otorhinolaryngol 2011;268:1593–6.

35. Fokkens WJ, Lund VJ, Mullol J, et al. European position paper on rhinosinusitis and nasal polyps 2012. Rhinol Suppl 2012;(23):1–298, 3 p preceding table of contents.

36. May A, Leone M, Afra J, et al. EFNS Guidelines on the treatment of cluster head-ache and other trigeminal autonomic cephalalgias. Eur J Neurol 2006;13(10): 1066–77.
37. Reid KI, Greene CS. Diagnosis and treatment of temporomandibular disorders: an ethical analysis of current practices. J Oral Rehabil 2013. http://dx.doi.org/10.1111/joor.12067.
38. Obermann M, Katsarava Z. Update on trigeminal neuralgia. Expert Rev Neurother 2009;9(3):323–9.
39. Evers S, Jensen R, European Federation of Neurological Societies. Treatment of medication overuse headache: guideline of the EFNS Headache Panel. Eur J Neurol 2011;18:1115–21.
40. Kari E, DelGaudio JM. Treatment of sinus headache as migraine: the diagnostic utility of triptans. Laryngoscope 2008;118:2235–9.
41. Dadgarnia MH, Atighechi A, Baradaranfar MH. The response to sodium valproate of patients with sinus headaches with normal endoscopic and CT findings. Eur Arch Otorhinolaryngol 2010;267:375–9.
42. Ishkanian G, Blumenthal H, Webster CJ, et al. Efficacy of sumatriptan tablets in migraineurs self-descibed or physician-diagnosed as having sinus headache: a randomized, double-blind, placebo-controlled study. Clin Ther 2007;29:99–109.
43. Novak VJ, Makek M. Pathogenesis and treatment of migraine and neurovascular headaches with rhinogenic trigger. Head Neck 1992;14:467–72.
44. Tosun F, Gerek M, Ozkaptan Y. Nasal surgery for contact point headaches. Head-ache 2000;40:237–40.
45. Welge-Luessen A, Hauser R, Schmid N, et al. Endonasal surgery for contact point headaches: a 10 year longitudinal study. Laryngoscope 2003;113:2151–6.
46. Yazici ZM, Cabalar M, Sayin I, et al. Rhinologic evaluation in patient with primary headache. J Craniofac Surg 2010;21:1688–91.

Red Flags and Comfort Signs for Ominous Secondary Headaches

Roger K. Cady, MD

KEYWORDS

- Headache • Secondary • Red flag • Comfort sign

KEY POINTS

- Secondary headaches are classified by the cause of the underlying disease process that is causing the headache.
- Maintaining a high level of vigilance and having a structured approach to evaluating all patients with headache is the key to timely diagnosis of secondary headache disorders.
- Diagnostic testing is indicated based on the suspected disorder and management is determined by treatment of the underlying disease causing the headache.

The number of disorders associated with the symptom of headache is as impressive as it is complex. Timely identification and diagnosis of secondary headaches often poses a significant challenge to clinicians. No single test or imaging study can conclusively diagnose all headache disorders. The most effective tool a clinician has to evaluate a patient with headache is a good history. Effective communication between a health care professional and patient is the essential key to successful diagnosis.

The consequences of missing a serious secondary headache can be severe.[1] However, a serious disorder as a cause of headache is uncommon, especially in the outpatient setting.[2] In medical settings such as emergency departments, referral centers, or urgent care facilities, the frequency of secondary headaches is higher,[3] but, even in these settings, secondary headaches are less common than primary headache disorders. Although this fact is comforting, it is often the familiarity with headache that is the reason a secondary disorder is sometimes overlooked. Therefore, it is essential that health care professionals maintain a high level of vigilance when evaluating a patient with headache, especially in patients with long-standing primary headache disorders. A secondary headache is likely to mimic a preexisting primary headache.[4] It has been estimated that approximately 90% of patients with a secondary headache also have a primary headache disorder and a normal examination.[5] Therefore, establishing a systematic approach to evaluating the patient with a complaint of headache is the best insurance against missing a disorder associated with serious secondary headaches.

Headache Care Center, 3805 South Kansas Expressway, Springfield, MO 65807, USA
E-mail address: rcady@headachecare.com

Otolaryngol Clin N Am 47 (2014) 289–299
http://dx.doi.org/10.1016/j.otc.2013.10.010

PRIMARY VERSUS SECONDARY HEADACHE

The first step in evaluating a patient with the complaint of headache is to differentiate primary from secondary headache. Primary headaches are syndromes in which headache is the disease process. They are classified according to symptoms.[2] The most common primary headache disorders are migraine, tension-type headache, and cluster headache. Less common primary headaches include other trigeminal autonomic cephalalgias; primary stabbing headache; headaches associated with cough, exertion, or sexual activity; new-onset persistent daily headache; and primary thunderclap headaches.[2] The common primary headaches are, by definition, recurrent and thus have generally been experienced by the patient on multiple occasions. The less common primary headaches are also usually recurrent (with the general exception of primary thunderclap headache), but these often require diagnostic work-up to exclude disorders. Only after repeated episodes of the same headache can the diagnosis of primary headache be firmly established.

Secondary headaches are classified by their causes. In secondary headaches, headache is a symptom of an underlying pathologic process. In general, secondary headaches are unfamiliar or new to the patient. The clinical caveat in this classification is that whenever a clinician is evaluating a new or different headache, there should be a high index of suspicion for a disorder. For diseases known to cause headache, the disorder often occurs in close temporal proximity to the onset of headache.[6]

Central to understanding the distinction between primary and secondary headaches is that symptoms alone are inadequate criteria for differentiating primary and secondary headaches. The brain has limited mechanisms to express pain. The symptoms included in diagnostic criteria of primary headache disorders are also frequently present in secondary headache disorders, and a patient can experience a secondary headache with the same symptoms as any primary headache disorder.[7,8] More often, it is the context in which a headache occurs that allows timely differentiation between primary and secondary headaches. The key element is for the clinician to accurately ascertain whether the evaluation is of a new or different type of headache, or whether it is an evaluation of an already established pattern of headache that is consistent and stable over time.

Consider the following case study: EM is a 42-year-old woman with a history of migraine of 30 years or more. Over the past 5 years, the migraines have occurred between 2 and 4 times per month. She has experienced a good sustained abortive response to oral sumatriptan for many years. She uses propranolol long acting 80 mg as migraine prophylaxis and to control hypertension. At an office visit 6 months ago, her migraine was well controlled and no changes were made in her treatment plan.

She presents stating that over the last 6 weeks her migraines have been getting worse. She reports that she has some type of headache almost every day and the migraines are worsening in intensity. The headaches are associated with nausea and sensory hypersensitivity, but the intensity of these symptoms varies from day to day and at times it is worse than in the past. She is perplexed about why her migraines are getting worse because she is not under increased stress and there is no change in her menstrual cycle. She noted that during her last menstrual period the migraine was only mild, which was unusual for her. She reports that sumatriptan is less effective and no longer aborts her migraine, although generally it still provides relief. Her sleep is disrupted by the headache and frequently she is nauseated in the morning. Her mood is stable and there have been no other changes in her health or medication usage. Her examination is normal.

Should this history sound alarm bells for the evaluating health care professional? Although the history alone does not diagnose a specific disorder, it does provide reasons for a high index of suspicion to evaluate this patient further. Most significant in this history is that the patient is communicating a change in her headache pattern that is distinct from her established primary headache disorder. Thus further evaluation of a headache in evolution is warranted. Although this change in headache pattern may be a progression of her migraine, there is little support in her history for this rapid transformation into a new headache pattern. In addition, her long-recognized response to sumatriptan has changed and she specifically noted that during menses this headache was different than her usual migraine. This patient should be evaluated for a secondary headache disorder.

The boundaries that define primary and secondary headaches are often indistinct and require a clinician to take time and care in interpreting a patient's history and to sift astutely through the hundreds of patients presenting with primary headache in order not to overlook the rare patient with a serious disorder. Again, the most valuable tool for accomplishing proper diagnosis is effective communication with the patient.

TAKING A HEADACHE HISTORY

Making a headache diagnosis is often considered an exercise in quizzing a patient with a checklist of headache characteristics and associated symptoms. Some questions are common to any textbook discussion of headache history, such as: where is the headache located? What is its intensity? What is the quality of the pain? What are the specific symptoms associated with the headache? What are the exacerbating and alleviating factors for the headache? However, primary and secondary headaches share symptom expression and thus symptoms alone are of limited value in defining secondary headache disorders.

A more effective strategy to obtain a good history is to let patients tell their stories by asking open-ended questions and considering the patient interview as a collaborative exercise between 2 experts: the clinician by virtue of education and medical experience, the patient by virtue of insightful understanding of the personal history.[9,10] Detailed questioning can be used by the clinician to elaborate specific aspects of the patient's history. In this way the headache history is put into a context that permits better differentiation and alignment of headache diagnoses and potential causes.

Key features to communicate and discuss can be summarized in the mnemonic of the 5 Ps: pattern, phenotype, patient, pharmacology, and precipitants or provoking factors.[11]

THE 5 PS
Pattern

Understanding the temporal pattern of headache is one of the most important elements of taking a headache history. The headache pattern reflects how the headaches have evolved over time and provides useful insight into important and sometimes subtle changes in an underlying headache pattern. A pattern that cannot be defined or is of recent onset is suspicious for a disorder, whereas a well-established stable pattern of headache indicates primary headaches. Querying about the pattern of headaches is also useful in detecting important changes such as chronification of migraine secondary to medication overuse. If changes in the pattern of a patient's headaches are not readily explained, or whenever the evaluation is of a new or recent headache, diagnostic evaluation for secondary headaches should be undertaken.

Phenotype

The phenotype of the headache refers to the characteristics and symptoms that are associated with the headache. Phenotypes may have recognizable diagnostic patterns such as migraine, tension-type headache, cluster headache, or other primary headaches, but headache with a recognizable primary headache phenotype does not ensure diagnostic exclusion of secondary headache. Different headache disorders can produce headache phenotypes mimicking any of the primary headache disorders. However, changes in a patient's headache phenotypes are an important means of differentiating primary and secondary headache. For example, it is reasonable to consider secondary headaches if a patient has been experiencing migraine with aura for years and suddenly develops tension-type headache without aura. A change in headache phenotype should be considered a red flag or warning sign. The presentation of a new headache phenotype should alert the clinician to a disorder, because accurate diagnosis of primary headache can only be made after repeated episodes of the same headache phenotype over time. Although not every red flag is the basis for exhaustive testing, it is the basis for additional diagnostic vigilance.

Patient Factors

Evaluation of patient factors is often overlooked as a critical aspect in evaluating a patient with headache. Critical patient factors include (1) age and general health; (2) baseline function before the onset of this headache; (3) return of the nervous system to its normal physiologic baseline function between each headache episode; (4) changes in normal physical, neurologic, or psychosocial function since the advent of this specific headache.

In addition, inquiry into the state of a patient's general health allows the clinician to probe for underlying diseases that may relate to secondary headache disorders. Questions relevant from this perspective concern (1) recent travel, both domestic and abroad; (2) recent trauma; (3) other medical diagnoses that may have a bearing on the headaches; (4) a family history to determine the risk of secondary headaches; (5) significant psychopathology; (6) reproductive status.

Pharmacology

An accurate accounting of recent pharmacologic interventions is a critical step in evaluating all patients with headache. Medications can cause headache, alter headache-related symptoms, or change important physiologic parameters such as cognitive function, body temperature, or blood pressure. It is essential to obtain a listing of prescription as well as nonprescription medications and to understand how and why specific mediations are being used (or not used). In addition, consider the possibility of recreational drug use and weigh the value of a drug screen.

Precipitating/Provoking Factors

The role of precipitating or provoking factors for secondary headaches includes evaluating risks associated with underlying disease such as infection, hypertension, pregnancy, coronary heart disease, or human immunodeficiency virus (HIV). Also, specific triggers are important to consider, such as trauma, exertion, sexual activity, or activities associated with a Valsalva maneuver. However, as headache frequency increases it is more difficult to assign specific triggers because at some point virtually any change seems to provoke the next headache. In addition, medications or food substances such as monosodium glutamate or tyramine, especially in the context of a monoamine oxidase inhibitor, may relate to the cause of a new secondary headache.

By incorporating the 5 Ps as a routine part of the history-taking process, a clinician can obtain a comprehensive understanding of both the headache and the patient experiencing the headache. From this vantage point, suspicion of a secondary disorder can be better ascertained and appropriate diagnostic testing initiated.

Physical Examination

Headache is a neurologic symptom, but numerous neurologic and non-neurologic diseases can cause secondary headache disorders. It is therefore essential to conduct both a thorough physical and neurologic examination. Components include vital signs with particular attention to blood pressure, weight change, and temperature. Examination of the mental status can often be made through the process of history taking. It is useful to examine nasal and oral cavities and perform a funduscopic examination. Examination of the thyroid, lungs, heart, and abdomen, as well as checking for lymphadenopathy, is also useful. While performing screening dermatologic and rheumatological examinations, look for inflammatory disease, rashes, signs of trauma or physical abuse, or evidence of intravenous drug use. In many instances, the history provides information indicating where to focus specific attention during the physical examination.

DIAGNOSTIC TESTING
Imaging Studies

Magnetic resonance imaging (MRI) is generally the preferred imaging modality for vascular disease, neoplastic disease, infections, intracranial hypotension, and rare encephalopathies (cerebral autosomal dominate arteriopathy with subcortical infarcts and leukoencephalopathy [CADASIL], mitochondrial encephalopathy, lactic acidosis, and strokelike [MELAS]). Computed tomography (CT) is preferred for suspected fractures, acute intracranial hemorrhages, paranasal disease, and mastoid disease. Magnetic resonance angiography (MRA) is indicated for vasculitis, arteriovenous malformations, pulsatile tinnitus, or dissection of the carotid or vertebral artery, and magnetic resonance venography is indicated for cavernous vein thrombosis.

Laboratory Testing

Laboratory evaluations may be useful in evaluation of a secondary headache and are determined by the suspected disorder. These include complete blood count, polymerase chain reaction, and blood and spinal fluid cultures to rule out central nervous system (CNS) infection or systemic disease. Thyroid testing, sedimentation rate, C-reactive protein (CRP), and coagulation studies should also be considered in specific circumstances. Pregnancy test and urinalysis may be important to diagnose headaches associated with pregnancy, especially toxemia. Serology and immunespecific testing for tick-borne diseases may be indicated in specific clinical settings. Genetic testing is indicated for rare headache disorders such as CADASIL and MELAS. Special procedures such as nasal endoscopy and a formal ophthalmologic examination are indicated when a nasal disorder or ocular disorder (particularly papilledema) is suspected.

Warning Signs, Caution Signs, and Comfort Signs

Information acquired through the history and physical examination is useful to identify specific factors that indicate primary or secondary headache disorders. This information can be used to target diagnostic testing or allay a patient's anxiety. For example, a patient who has episodes of headache in several different locations is unlikely to have a brain tumor or fixed vascular disorder, and people who are able to observe their visual auras with their eyes closed are unlikely to have ocular disease. **Table 1** shows

Table 1
Common warning signs and comfort factors that help differentiate primary and secondary headaches

Red Flags/Warning Signs	Comfort Signs
Abrupt onset of headache	Established stable pattern of
○ CNS hemorrhage	headache >6 mo
○ Reversible cerebral vasoconstriction	Variability of headache location
syndrome	Long-standing history of similar headache
○ Mass lesion	Exacerbation with menses
New headache pattern when	Return to baseline function between
≤5 y old	headaches
○ Systemic infection	Positive family history of primary headache
○ Congenital anomalies	disorder
≥50 y old	Normal physical and neurologic examination
○ Tumor	Consistently triggered by
○ Giant cell arteritis	○ Hormonal cycle
New onset or change in existing headache	○ Specific foods
pattern	○ Specific sensory input
○ Medication overuse	■ Light
○ Mass lesion	■ Odors
○ CNS infection	○ Weather changes
Neurologic signs or symptoms	
○ Mass lesion; primary or metastatic	
○ CNS infection	
○ Connective tissue disease	
○ Intracranial hypertension	
Head or neck trauma	
○ Hemorrhage	
○ Dissection	
Fever	
○ Systemic infection	
○ Meningoencephalitis	
○ Tick borne diseases especially with history	
of joint inflammation	
Weight loss	
○ Malignancy	
○ Systemic disease	
○ HIV	
Systemic disease	
○ HIV	
○ Inflammatory rheumatological disease	
○ Hypertensive crisis	
Pregnancy	
○ Toxemia	
○ Pituitary apoplexy	
Headaches triggered by exertion, sexual	
activity, cough, or Valsalva	
○ Mass lesion	
○ Subarachnoid hemorrhage	
○ Vertebral or carotid dissection	
Postural headaches	
○ Lumbar puncture headache	
○ Intracranial hypotension	

a list of common warning signs and comfort factors that help differentiate primary and secondary headaches.

ASSIGNING THE CAUSALITY OF A HEADACHE TO A DISORDER

The presence of a disorder does not confirm the cause of a secondary headache disorder. An incidental disorder is often discovered during a patient's work-up for headache and can become the focus of extensive medical evaluations and procedures. At times this can result in iatrogenic disease. As a precautionary note, it is worthwhile to question the causal relationship between the symptom of headache and the presence of a benign or insignificant disorder.

Factors useful in assigning causality include the temporal profile of an event, known association of specific disorders with headache, and the occurrence of headache or resolution of headache with treatment of the underlying disorder. None of these approaches is perfect and assigning causality requires astute clinical judgment. For example, providing an antibiotic for a patient with sinus migraine is associated with resolution of the headache, but so too would be an oral triptan. Because patients are often eager to accept a disorder as an explanation for their headaches, it is important to differentiate the presence of a disorder from the cause of the headache. Remember that invasive exploration for disease or assigning the causality of a disorder to symptoms may have unwanted consequences for the patient.

THE IMPORTANCE OF FOLLOW-UP EXAMINATION

One of the underappreciated aspects of managing a patient with headache is reevaluation of the patient over time. Timing of the evaluation is based on the disorder being considered. For example, a patient suspected of a CNS infection or trauma requires revaluation within minutes to hours, whereas reevaluation of a subtle neurologic sign may be accomplished over days or weeks. However, reevaluation of a patient with headaches can be a fruitful and effective diagnostic tool.

OMINOUS RED FLAGS

Red flags refer to specific warning signs or clinical circumstances in which the symptom of headache needs to be diagnosed quickly because it may represent the presence of a sinister disorder. Ominous red flags are shown in **Table 1** and include onset of new or different headache, abrupt onset of headache, headaches associated with trauma, onset of headache during pregnancy, and headache with fever or significant hypertension.

Ominous Headaches Associated with Abrupt Onset

Intense headache of abrupt onset may indicate subarachnoid hemorrhage (SAH). It is estimated that 25% of thunderclap headaches are secondary to subarachnoid hemorrhage.[12] Often patients state that SAHs are the worst headaches of their lives or describe the headache onset as like being hit with a bat. The outcome for patients with SAH is poor, with mortalities between 40% and 50%, with significant morbidity occurring in approximately 50% of survivors. An estimated 10% to 20% of individuals sustaining an SAH die before arriving at the hospital.[13]

Thunderclap or abrupt-onset headaches that resolve or markedly improve even after a short time also require careful diagnostic attention. This presentation is common for an unruptured cerebral aneurysm and a so-called sentinel bleed.[14]

An abrupt-onset severe headache requires an urgent noncontrast CT. If normal, and no contraindications exist, a lumbar puncture should follow[15–17] because CT can be normal in the immediate hours after a CNS bleed.[18] It is also important to recall that the sensitivity of CT scans to detect a subarachnoid bleed is inversely related to the time elapsed between the onset of bleeding and obtaining the CT. Sensitivity to detect hemorrhage is estimated at 95% within 24 hours; 74% by day 3; 50% by day 7; and nearly 0% by day 21.[19]

Other abrupt-onset secondary headaches to consider are intracerebral hemorrhage, arteriovenous malformation, arterial dissection, cerebral venous thrombosis, acute hypertensive crisis, pituitary apoplexy, or acute vasoconstrictive syndromes.[19] Whenever there is sudden abrupt onset of headache, think of vascular disorders.

Ominous Headaches Associated with Trauma

Trauma resulting in hemorrhage or edema in the CNS can be a life-threatening emergency and consequently accurate diagnosis is essential. Included in the differential is epidural, subdural, subarachnoid, and intraparenchymal hemorrhage. Trauma can at time appear mild but, particularly if a patient is elderly, on anticoagulants, or presenting with impaired cognition or other neurologic signs, an evaluation for hemorrhage is critical. Also, dissection of the carotid or vertebral artery should be suspected with cervical trauma, particularly in the presence of headache with neurologic symptoms such as Horner syndrome, dysarthria, dysphagia, or unsteadiness of gait.

Ominous Headaches Associated with CNS Infections

Infections of the CNS can have severe consequences including death. Prompt diagnosis and treatment are therefore paramount whenever an infectious cause is considered. Patients who are immunosuppressed are at particular risk and may present with few signs and symptoms of infectious disease. Children and the elderly are other populations at risk and treatment should be initiated as soon as possible, often pending completion of diagnostic testing. Headaches associated with fever and nuchal rigidity should be considered infectious until proved otherwise.

Ominous Headaches in Patients More than 50 Years of Age

Onset of headache after 50 years of age should be considered a warning sign for secondary headache. The most ominous secondary headache in this patient group is arguably giant cell arteritis (GCA; temporal arteritis) because without prompt administration of steroids it can lead to permanent blindness. GCA is a systemic disease and often there are associated symptoms and signs such as weight loss, malaise, fever, scalp tenderness, diplopia, or jaw claudication.[20] GCA is more common in women than men and is most often seen in patients older than 50 years, with a mean age at diagnosis of 70 years.[21] A sedimentation rate and CRP followed by a temporal artery biopsy should be considered on all patients presenting with a new headache after 50 years of age. When a biopsy is performed, a sufficient length of the artery must be biopsied, because so-called skip area can occur in GCA, resulting in false-negative results.[22] High-dose steroids should be initiated pending biopsy results.

Other important secondary headaches presenting after 50 years of age are primary and metastatic brain tumors and cerebrovascular disease.

HYPERTENSIVE CRISIS AND HEADACHE

A hypertensive crisis is defined as rapid increase in blood pressure with a systolic pressure greater than 180 mm Hg and diastolic reading greater than 120 mm Hg.

Common symptoms include severe headache often with mental confusion and blurred vision, chest pain, epistasis, nausea and vomiting, dyspnea, seizure, and anxiety. A hypertensive crisis can lead to stroke, pulmonary edema, myocardial infarction, arterial rupture outside the CNS, and encephalopathy.[23] It is more common in African American men, young adults, and during pregnancy (toxemia).[24] It may be idiopathic or related to underlying hypertension. Other causes to consider are medication, medication interactions, illicit drugs, or (less commonly) a pheochromocytoma.[25]

OMINOUS HEADACHES ASSOCIATED WITH PREGNANCY AND THE POSTPARTUM PERIOD

In general, primary headaches, particularly migraine, tend to improve during pregnancy.[26] Headache with onset during pregnancy or in the postpartum period needs to be evaluated carefully. After 20 weeks, headache associated with hypertension and proteinuria is likely secondary to preeclampsia or toxemia. If seizures occur, it becomes eclampsia.[27] Both are medical emergencies. Also, preexisting migraine with aura is a risk for stroke during pregnancy, especially in the setting of coagulation defects.

In the postpartum period, pituitary infarction (pituitary apoplexy) can occur and clinicians should also consider postspinal headache if a woman was provided with epidural analgesia and complains of a postural headache.

Secondary Headaches: Important but Less Ominous

Medication overuse headache

Numerous medications have been implicated in maintaining and worsening primary headache disorders, and particularly migraine. Medication overuse headache (MOH) is a clinical diagnosis, whereas medication overuse is a consensus diagnosis based on specific quantities of abortive medications (**Box 1**). MOH is diagnosed when the underlying primary headache disorder is associated with increasing use and diminishing benefit of abortive medications. The medication causing the headache needs to be discontinued.

Orthostatic headaches

Orthostatic headaches are characterized by a moderate to severe headache that occurs when a person is vertical and that improves when supine. They indicate a cerebral

---

Box 1
International Headache Society diagnostic criteria for headache attributed to a substance or its withdrawal

8.2. MOH

    A. Headache occurring on greater than or equal to 15 days per month in a patient with a preexisting headache disorder

    B. Regular overuse for more than 3 months of one or more drugs that can be taken for acute and/or symptomatic treatment of headache

    C. Not better accounted for by another International Classification of Headache Disorders, Third Edition (ICHD-3) diagnosis.

From Headache Classification Committee of the International Headache Society (IHS). The international classification of headache disorders, 3rd edition (beta version). Cephalalgia 2013;33(9):733; with permission.

spinal fluid leak that can be spontaneous or related to traumatic events such as a spinal tap. More rarely they occur without a cerebrospinal fluid leak. They may be diagnosed with the aid of MRI showing pachymeningeal enhancement with gadolinium or radioisotope cisternography.

SUMMARY

Secondary headaches are classified by the cause of the underlying disease process that is causing the headache. There are hundreds of secondary headache diagnoses and this article is not an exhaustive discussion of secondary headache disorders. Maintaining a high level of vigilance and having a structured approach to evaluating all patients with headache is the key to timely diagnosis of secondary headache disorders. Diagnostic testing is indicated based on the suspected disorder and management is determined by treatment of the underlying disease causing the headache.

REFERENCES

1. Headache Classification Committee of the International Headache Society (IHS). The International Classification of Headache Disorders, 3rd edition (beta version). Cephalalgia 2013;33(9):629–808.
2. Dodick DW. Clinical clues and clinical rules: primary vs. secondary headache. Adv Stud Med 2003;3(6C):S550–5.
3. Martin VT. The diagnostic evaluation of secondary headache disorders. Headache 2011;51(2):346–52.
4. Crystal SC, Robbins MS. Tension-type headache mimics. Curr Pain Headache Rep 2011;15(6):459–66.
5. Dodick DW. Pearls: headache. Semin Neurol 2010;30(1):74–81.
6. Heinze A, Heinze-Kuhn K, Göbel H. Classification of headache disorders. Schmerz 2007;21(3):263–73.
7. Schankin CJ, Straube A. Secondary headaches: secondary or still primary? J Headache Pain 2012;13(4):263–70.
8. Ravishankar K. Optimising primary headache management. J Assoc Physicians India 2006;54:928–34.
9. Lipton RB, Cady RK, Farmer K, et al. Managing migraine: a healthcare professional's guide to collaborative migraine care. Hamilton (Ontario): Baxter Publishing; 2008.
10. Cady RK, Lipton RB, Farmer K, et al. Managing migraine: a patient's guide to successful migraine care. Hamilton (Ontario): Baxter Publishing; 2008.
11. Hutchinson S, Cady RK. Chronic migraine: making the diagnosis. Primary Issues. September 11, 2011. Available at: http://www.primaryissues.org. Accessed October 28, 2013.
12. Landtblom AM, Fridriksson S, Boivie J, et al. Sudden onset headache: a prospective study of features, incidence and causes. Cephalalgia 2002;22(5):354–60.
13. van Gijn J, Kerr RS, Rinkel GJ. Subarachnoid haemorrhage. Lancet 2007; 369(9558):306–18.
14. de Falco FA. Sentinel headache. Neurol Sci 2004;25(Suppl 3):S215–7.
15. Stewart H, Reuben A, McDonald J. LP or not LP, that is the question: gold standard or unnecessary procedure in subarachnoid haemorrhage? Emerg Med J 2013. [Epub ahead of print].
16. Edlow JA, Caplan LR. Avoiding pitfalls in the diagnosis of subarachnoid hemorrhage. N Engl J Med 2000;342(1):29–36.

17. Fine B, Singh N, Aviv R, Macdonald RL. Decisions: does a patient with a thunderclap headache need a lumbar puncture? CMAJ 2012;184(5):555–6.
18. Laughlin S, Montanera W. Central nervous system imaging. When is CT more appropriate than MRI? Postgrad Med 1998;104(5):73–6.
19. De Luca GC, Bartleson JD. When and how to investigate the patient with headache. Semin Neurol 2010;30(2):131–44.
20. Ness T, Bley TA, Schmidt WA, Lamprecht P. The diagnosis and treatment of giant cell arteritis. Dtsch Arztebl Int 2013;110(21):376–85.
21. Wall M, Corbett JJ. Arteritis. In: Olesen J, Goadsby PJ, Ramadan NM, et al, editors. The headaches. 3rd edition. Philadelphia: Lippincott Williams & Wilkins; 2006. p. 901.
22. Klein RG, Campbell RJ, Hunder GG, Carney JA. Skip lesions in temporal arteritis. Mayo Clin Proc 1976;51:504–10.
23. Rodriguez MA, Kumar SK, De Caro M. Hypertensive crisis. Cardiol Rev 2010; 18(2):102–7.
24. Badr KF, Brenner BM. Vascular injury to the kidney. In: Fauci A, Kasper D, Longo DL, et al, editors. Harrison's principals of internal medicine. 17th edition. New York: McGraw Hill; 2008. p. 1813.
25. Frank J, Sommerfeld D. Clinical approach in treatment of resistant hypertension. Integr Blood Press Control 2009;2:9–23.
26. Kvisvik EV, Stovner LJ, Helde G, Bovim G, Linde M. Headache and migraine during pregnancy and puerperium: the MIGRA-study. J Headache Pain 2011;12: 443–51.
27. Cipolla MJ, Kraig RP. Seizures in women with preeclampsia: mechanisms and management. Fetal Matern Med Rev 2011;22:91–108.

The Essential Role of the Otolaryngologist in the Diagnosis and Management of Temporomandibular Joint and Chronic Oral, Head, and Facial Pain Disorders

Howard A. Israel, DDS[a,b,*], Laura J. Davila, DDS[a]

KEYWORDS

- Temporomandibular joint • Chronic oral, facial and head pain • Otalgia
- TMJ arthroscopy • TMJ exercise • Passive motion jaw rehabilitation
- Temporomandibular disorders

KEY POINTS

- Chronic oral, head, and facial pain (COHFP) disorders are frequently misdiagnosed, therefore a constant reevaluation of the diagnosis and response to treatment is required.
- Otologic symptoms are often caused by temporomandibular disorders (TMDs), and a careful history and clinical examination are the most important factors in making an accurate diagnosis and appropriate referral.
- Joint overload and lack of motion lead to pathologic changes resulting in inflammatory and degenerative temporomandibular joint disease.
- Principles for treating inflammatory and degenerative temporomandibular joint disorders are to reduce load, increase mobility with passive motion, reduce inflammation and muscle spasm, and manage pain.
- For patients with severe temporomandibular joint disorders that fail to improve with appropriate treatment, the least invasive procedure to treat the pathologic condition and improve function is indicated.

Portions of this review were updated from: Israel H. The essential role of the oral and maxillofacial surgeon in the diagnosis, management, causation and prevention of chronic orofacial pain: clinical perspectives. In: Fonseca RJ, editor. Oral and maxillofacial surgery. 2nd edition. St. Louis, Missouri: Elsevier Health Sciences; 2009. p. 132–55.

[a] Division of Dentistry Oral & Maxillofacial Surgery, Weill-Cornell Medical College, New York Presbyterian Hospital, Cornell University, 525 East 68th Street, New York, NY 10065, USA; [b] Columbia University College of Dental Medicine, 630 West 168th Street, New York, NY 10032, USA
* Corresponding author. 12 Bond Street, Great Neck, NY 11021.
E-mail address: drhowardisrael@yahoo.com

Otolaryngol Clin N Am 47 (2014) 301–331
http://dx.doi.org/10.1016/j.otc.2013.12.001
0030-6665/14/$ – see front matter © 2014 Elsevier Inc. All rights reserved.

INTRODUCTION

In 1934, Costen[1] published a paper in the *Annals of Otology, Rhinology and Laryngology* on "A Syndrome of Ear and Sinus Symptoms Dependent on Disturbed Function of the Temporomandibular Joint." Costen observed patients with ear, jaw, and sinus pain and theorized that an altered occlusion resulted in temporomandibular joint disease as the major etiologic factor. Furthermore, he recommended correction of the occlusion to relieve pressure on the temporomandibular joint and surrounding structures, ultimately leading to resolution of the symptoms. Thus, the importance of the specialty of otolaryngology in the diagnosis and treatment of oral, head, and face pain was reinforced 80 years ago and continues to this day. Although Costen's proposal that an altered occlusion was the main cause of head and facial pain has been refuted by evidence-based research, to his credit, he did understand that the site and source of complex head and facial pain are often not the same. Today, 8 decades after the introduction of Costen syndrome, there are many clinicians who still treat patients according to the observations of Dr Costen in 1934.

The diagnosis and management of COHFP has been a subject of great controversy over the years and continues to this day. This situation is unfortunate, because there have been great advances in our understanding of these conditions based on solid research over the past 25 years.

Common clinical scenarios that the otolaryngologist is presented with include the following:

1. Patients with severe persistent ear pain with negative otologic findings who have inflammatory temporomandibular joint disease.
2. Patients with COHFP and masticatory dysfunction who are ultimately diagnosed with neoplasia or other serious disorders (eg, trigeminal neuralgia, temporal arteritis).
3. Patients with oropharyngeal cancers treated with surgery and radiation leading to trismus because of radiation fibrosis, making early detection of recurrent or second primary cancers extremely difficult if not impossible for the clinician.
4. Patients with persistent maxillary dental pain, undergoing multiple dental procedures that fail to reduce symptoms (eg. extractions, root canal therapy) who eventually are diagnosed with acute or chronic maxillary sinusitis.
5. Patients with tinnitus symptoms, resistant to treatment, and coexisting TMDs.

This article clarifies the current state of knowledge of COHFP conditions with the inclusion of temporomandibular joint disorders as just one component of the variety of conditions that can cause head and facial pain. Obtaining an accurate diagnosis in a timely manner is extremely important because COHFP symptoms can be caused by a variety of pathologic conditions that can be inflammatory, degenerative, neurologic, neoplastic, or systemic in origin. The essential role of the specialty of otolaryngology in the diagnosis and management of patients with these complex COHFP conditions is emphasized.

PITFALLS LEADING TO MISDIAGNOSIS OF COHFP

The reasons for the difficulty in properly diagnosing COHFP and TMDs are multifactorial. The following factors that can lead to misdiagnosis are important for the clinician to be aware:

1. Complex regional anatomy of the head and neck, often resulting in disparity between the site and the source of pain.

2. Symptoms of pain, limitation of mandibular movement, joint noise, tinnitus, and altered occlusion are not specific for the pathologic condition. Thus, these symptoms can be caused by local otologic and temporomandibular joint disorders or infectious, neoplastic, neurologic, and systemic conditions.
3. Chronic tissue damage from trauma and/or multiple surgical procedures can lead to central sensitization of sensory nerve pathways, leading to neuropathic pain, allodynia (pain response to nonpainful stimuli), and hyperalgesia (excessive pain response to mildly painful stimuli). The presence of neuropathic pain can make accurate diagnosis extremely difficult because the clinician can easily be misled into believing that the source of the pain is localized, when in fact, there is a central-nervous-system-mediated component.

The following case scenarios are provided to demonstrate common clinical situations that can potentially lead to misdiagnosis of COHFP and TMDs.

Inflammatory/Degenerative Temporomandibular Joint Disorders Initially Presenting with Symptoms of Otalgia

A major factor contributing to confusion between otologic pathology and temporomandibular joint pathology is close anatomic proximity and common sensory innervation via the auriculotemporal nerve. Patients often cannot differentiate ear pain from temporomandibular joint pain, and thus, otologic pathology may cause temporomandibular joint pain and temporomandibular joint pathology may cause otologic pain.

CASE REPORT #1: TEMPOROMANDIBULAR JOINT SYNOVITIS AND OTALGIA

A 26-year-old woman presented to the otolaryngologist with severe right-sided ear pain for the past 9 months. The patient reported having an upper respiratory tract infection 9 months ago and after the resolution of the respiratory infection, developed persistent right-sided ear pain. She also noticed that chewing made her symptoms worse and that there was limitation in her jaw opening. The otologic examination and audiometric findings were normal. Palpation of the anterior aspect of the right external auditory canal revealed significant tenderness, compared to the right. The maximum interincisal mandibular opening distance was measured at 20 mm with deviation to the right and produced severe pain in the right ear (**Fig. 1A**). The patient was unable to shift her jaw to the left because of severe pain in the right ear. The patient was given a tongue blade to bite on, and this produced severe pain in the right ear. The otolaryngologist concluded that the diagnosis was a temporomandibular joint disorder. The recommended course of action was ibuprofen, 600 mg, thrice daily and for the patient to be evaluated by an oral and maxillofacial surgeon with expertise in the diagnosis and management of temporomandibular joint disorders.

The patient was evaluated by an oral and maxillofacial surgeon who diagnosed her with right temporomandibular joint synovitis, masticatory muscle spasm with a clenching habit, as a major etiologic factor. A night guard oral appliance was fabricated to attempt to reduce the forces of nocturnal clenching. The patient was instructed to perform passive jaw motion exercises thrice daily. She was continued on ibuprofen, 600 mg, thrice daily and prescribed diazepam, 5 mg, to be taken at bedtime to help to reduce stress and act as a muscle relaxant. After using the oral appliance for 1 week, the patient's symptoms increased, with further exacerbation of the right-sided ear pain. The patient returned to the otolaryngologist who noted severe pain on palpation over the right temporomandibular joint as well as in the external auditory canal. Although examination of the middle ear with an otoscope did cause pain, the tympanic membrane and middle ear examination was unremarkable. The maximum interincisal opening distance was now 15 mm, and the patient was unable to occlude her teeth properly on the right side because the upper and lower posterior teeth were not meeting. The otolaryngologist and the oral and maxillofacial surgeon conferred, and the patient was diagnosed with an acute temporomandibular joint synovitis. The patient was placed on a 1-week oral steroid medication with a tapering dose and was referred back to the oral and maxillofacial surgeon for further management.

The clinical findings were essentially unchanged when the patient was seen by the oral and maxillofacial surgeon. The pain level was rated as 9 on the visual analog scale (0, no pain; 10, the most severe pain); the maximum interincisal opening distance was measured at 18 mm with deviation to the right and causing severe pain localized to the right ear and temporomandibular joint region. The left lateral excursion of the mandible was severely limited to 3 mm and caused pain in the right temporomandibular joint. The right lateral excursion was 10 mm and did not exacerbate pain. The occlusion was class I with a 1-mm right-sided posterior open bite. Mild manipulation of the mandible to attempt to position the right posterior teeth to occlude caused severe right-sided temporomandibular joint and ear pain. The left temporomandibular joint was nonpainful and had normal rotational and translational movement. A panoramic radiograph was obtained, which was unremarkable. Temporomandibular joint magnetic resonance imaging (MRI) was performed, which revealed anterior disk displacement without reduction of both the right and left temporomandibular joints. A significant finding was a large effusion in the right temporomandibular joint superior joint space as demonstrated by enhanced white signal intensity on the T2 images (see **Fig. 1B**). The clinical examination and MRI findings were consistent with a right temporomandibular joint synovitis. The patient was frustrated having had this problem for 9 months without any significant resolution in spite of a full course of nonsurgical management.

The oral and maxillofacial surgeon recommended right temporomandibular joint arthroscopic surgery, which was performed under sedation and local anesthesia. This surgery revealed a severe grade 4 synovitis of the posterior synovial tissues as well as adhesions in the superior joint space (see **Fig. 1C**). Operative arthroscopy was performed, which involved lysis of adhesions and removal with a motorized minishaver and a 2.0 mm full radius blade. Areas of significant synovitis were localized, and under direct vision, betamethasone (6 mg/mL) was injected with a #25 gauge spinal needle. The disk was mobilized with a graded probe instrument. After the arthroscopic surgery, the patient was placed on nonsteroidal antiinflammatory drugs, muscle relaxants, and a nonchew diet for 3 weeks. Most importantly, passive motion exercises to gradually stretch the mandible open to restore normal range of motion were started immediately. The passive motion exercise sessions were performed for 15 minutes thrice daily. Three weeks after the arthroscopic surgery, the maximum interincisal opening distance was 38 mm and the pain level was reduced to 3 with maximum opening. At rest, without jaw movement, there was no ear or temporomandibular joint pain. The diet was gradually advanced, and at 3 months postoperatively, the maximum interincisal opening distance was 41 mm, the pain level on the visual analog scale was 1, and the patient was able to chew on soft foods. She continued performing her passive motion exercises twice daily. At 1 year postoperatively, the patient has no pain at rest and occasional pain levels of up to 2 with maximum opening. The patient is able to chew on almost all foods, although she avoids very chewy foods such as bagels and hero sandwiches.

Discussion Case #1

A common scenario is a patient who seeks consultation with an otolaryngologist regarding the onset of acute ear pain or the persistence of chronic ear pain. When the clinical findings do not support an otologic cause, the patient is often referred for evaluation of a temporomandibular joint disorder. The patient may seek multiple opinions from otolaryngologists, neurologists, dentists, and oral and maxillofacial surgeons in a quest for appropriate diagnosis and treatment. The importance of establishing an accurate diagnosis cannot be over emphasized because it is essential for proper treatment. Thus, failure to establish the diagnosis will often result in persistent symptoms or inappropriate treatments. In spite of this, the astute clinician can use the following guidelines to help differentiate pathologic conditions of the ear versus those of the temporomandibular joint:

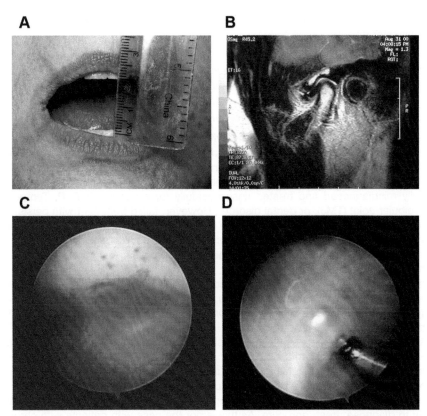

Fig. 1. (A) 26-year-old with severe right-sided ear pain, increased pain due to jaw movement, limited jaw opening of 20 mm with deviation to the painful side. (B) MRI of the right temporomandibular joint demonstrates a synovial effusion on the T2 images with fluid in the superior joint space. Anterior disk position is also present. (C, D) Arthroscopy of the right temporomandibular joint demonstrated grade 4 synovitis and adhesions of the posterior recess. Inflammation of the synovial membrane with associated adhesions area significant tissue changes that cause pain and limitation in joint mobility.

1. Temporomandibular joint pathology is generally increased by mandibular movement and function.
2. If the pain is increased significantly because of chewing (or biting firmly on a tongue blade during the initial examination), it often indicates a temporomandibular joint or masticatory muscle disorder.
3. Temporomandibular joint pathology will often cause a restriction in the range of motion of the affected joint. Thus, a right temporomandibular joint disorder often causes the mandible to deviate to the right with attempts at maximum opening. Furthermore, when a patient attempts an opposite lateral excursion (for example, sliding the lower jaw to the left in the aforementioned scenario) there will be restricted movement and increased pain.
4. Temporomandibular joint noise (clicking or crepitus) does not necessarily indicate temporomandibular joint disease as the cause of the pain.
5. If the patient points directly to the temporomandibular joint as the location of the source of pain during attempts at maximum jaw opening, it usually indicates a temporomandibular joint disorder.

6. Patients who have excessive clenching habits will often have tender temporalis and masseter muscles on palpation.

Although none of the above guidelines are absolute, because there are always exceptions to the rule, these simple observations can give the clinician an important clue as to which direction the diagnostic workup should follow.

Neoplasia Misdiagnosed as COHFP and Temporomandibular Joint Disorders

The specialty of otolaryngology plays a vital role in educating other health professionals about the consequences of misdiagnosing serious neoplastic conditions with symptoms that mimic COFHP and temporomandibular joint disorders. Unfortunately, there are numerous examples of patients with COFHP symptoms who were initially misdiagnosed and treated unsuccessfully for a routine COFHP, Temporomandibular Joint (TMJ), or dental disorder. However, failed treatment with persistent symptoms must alert the clinician that the diagnosis may be faulty. There are serious consequences of continued failed treatment and misdiagnosis because this may lead to delayed diagnosis and treatment of a neoplastic process. An important rule for all clinicians to follow is as follows:

If the patient does not respond as expected to treatment based on the most likely diagnosis in one's differential diagnosis, then the clinician must reevaluate the diagnosis and rule out other conditions that may be causing the patient's symptoms.

The constant reevaluation of the diagnosis based on the patient's response to treatment is referred to as the Flexible Diagnoses-Management Concept. It is common, even for the experienced clinician, to be uncertain of the diagnosis and treatment of a patient with chronic orofacial pain, which is unlike the more common situation in which a patient with acute pain and swelling presents with an abscess that is generally easy to diagnose, treat, and cure. As this is not the case with patients with chronic pain, it is important for the clinician to have a different mind-set with the development of differential diagnoses that remain flexible. The concept here is that the clinician develops an initial differential diagnoses and treats the patient according to the most likely condition or conditions causing the chronic pain. Based on the response to treatment, there is a continual reevaluation of the diagnoses and treatment. Failure to constantly reevaluate the response to treatment and diagnosis can lead to serious consequences with misdiagnosis of lethal pathologic conditions that mimic COFHP and temporomandibular joint disorders.

Most importantly, the clinical presentation needs to be looked at carefully. Patients with jaw pain, limitation of mobility, and deviation of the mandible to one side on opening often have an intra-articular temporomandibular joint pathology. However, there are other pathologic conditions that can lead to deviation of the mandible. The motor branches of the fifth cranial nerve provide innervation to the muscles of mastication, including the masseter, temporalis, lateral, and medial pterygoid muscles. As the lateral pterygoid muscle attaches to the mandibular condyle and anterior capsule of the temporomandibular joint, it is responsible for translation of the temporomandibular joint. Lack of motor function of the lateral pterygoid muscle will cause failure of translation of the mandibular condyle during jaw opening movements, resulting in deviation of the mandible to the affected side because of the unopposed action of the lateral pterygoid muscle on the unaffected side. The clinician must be thorough and check for normal motor function of the muscles of mastication. Lack of muscle tone of the masseter, temporalis and lateral pterygoid muscles must alert the clinician to a fifth cranial nerve deficit as the cause of the mandibular deviation with opening.

Furthermore, once there is clear evidence of a cranial nerve deficit, the clinician must assume a diagnosis of neoplasia until proven otherwise.

Central lesions affecting the trigeminal ganglion often cause symptoms that are located in the peripheral distribution of the fifth cranial nerve (**Fig. 2**). Therefore, dental pain in the absence of objective evidence of local pathologic condition must be viewed with suspicion. Complicating the clinical picture is the fact that there are many painful dental conditions that do not manifest with clear objective clinical findings.

For example, a painful inflammation of the dental pulp caused by decay may not demonstrate any pathologic condition seen on radiographs, particularly if the patient has a metal crown on the tooth. Masticatory muscle pain from clenching also has negative radiographic findings. Therefore, once treatment of these conditions is initiated, it is extremely important to evaluate the patient's response to treatment. If the symptoms persist, it is necessary to reevaluate the diagnosis, and the clinician must consider the possibility of the local pain being caused by a central pathology.

Dental pain does not necessarily originate from the oral cavity. Central nervous system pathology can cause pain in the oral and maxillofacial region. There are numerous examples of dental pain treated by numerous clinicians without any relief because the pain was caused by a central nervous system lesion. A common condition that often presents with a history of numerous failed dental treatments is trigeminal neuralgia. A careful history reveals that the character of the pain is shocklike, usually unilateral and so severe that it stops the patient in the middle of a sentence. Although the pain is of high intensity, it is often short in duration (usually seconds) and there is often a trigger point that will suddenly bring on the severe pain with an innocuous stimulus. A light touch to the face, wind on the face, or brushing teeth is often the triggering stimulus for the severe pain from trigeminal neuralgia. Once the diagnosis is established, initial treatment is usually a course of anticonvulsant medication (eg. gabapentin, carbamazepine). It is extremely important for trigeminal neuralgia to be viewed as a symptom, and thus, a brain scan is necessary to determine if there is a central nervous system lesion compressing the trigeminal nerve. If medications fail to control the severe symptoms, the patient should be referred to a neurologic surgeon.

Another common scenario for the otolaryngologist is the patient with persist dental pain and failed dental treatment in the presence of maxillary sinusitis. Infection of the

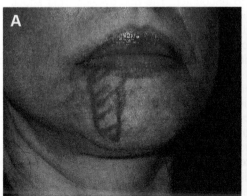 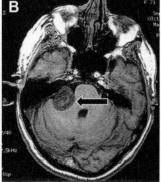

Fig. 2. (*A*) Patient with chronic right mandibular pain treated for 2 years with multiple failed dental treatments. The patient had paresthesia involving the right lower lip and chin. (*B*) MRI demonstrating an acoustic neuroma (*arrow*).

maxillary sinus will cause pain because of nociceptive stimulation of the posterior, middle, and anterior superior divisions of the maxillary nerve (V2). These sensory nerves are also stimulated when there is dental pathology of the maxillary posterior teeth, and therefore, patients with maxillary sinusitis often complain of severe tooth pain with dental interventions failing to resolve symptoms (**Fig. 3**).

The clinician must be aware of systemic pathologic conditions that can cause temporomandibular and oral, facial, and head pain. Conditions such as fibromyalgia, rheumatoid arthritis, psoriasis, and osteoarthritis can affect the temporomandibular joint and the surrounding muscles of mastication causing severe symptoms. Patients with multiple sclerosis are more prone to trigeminal neuralgia. If there is a history of herpes zoster, facial pain can occur because of postherpetic neuralgia. Cardiac ischemia is also a common cause of facial pain. The pain may occur in the throat, mandible, temporomandibular joint, and teeth. Approximately 32% of patients with cardiac ischemia had craniofacial pain along with other cardiac symptoms. One study revealed that craniofacial pain was the only complaint in 6% of individuals with cardiac ischemia.[2] As cardiac ischemia and acute myocardial infarction require immediate referral and management, the implications for the treating clinician are significant.

TEMPOROMANDIBULAR JOINT AND MASTICATORY MUSCLE DISORDERS: CURRENT CONCEPTS OF DIAGNOSIS AND MANAGEMENT

Perhaps one of the most common of the COHFP disorders that causes otologic symptoms without otologic pathology is the group of disorders encompassing inflammatory/degenerative temporomandibular joint disease as well as disorders of the muscles of mastication. TMD is an extremely broad and nonspecific diagnostic term, encompassing both joint and muscle disorders of the masticatory system. To specify whether a diagnosis is primarily intra-articular (coming directly from the temporomandibular joint) or primarily extra-articular (coming from structures outside the temporomandibular joint) is far more useful in patient management.

Other extra-articular conditions beyond the common masticatory muscle disorders can mimic temporomandibular joint disease, for example, coronoid hyperplasia, neoplasia, deep space infections, and myositis ossificans. Here the authors focus on the most common temporomandibular joint and masticatory muscle conditions that the clinician is likely to encounter. The abbreviation TMJ should be avoided and, when used, should refer solely to the anatomic structure. The term TMJ is often inappropriately used by patients and some health professionals to include the variety of disorders of the musculoskeletal component of the head and neck affecting the temporomandibular joint and surrounding masticatory muscles.

Temporomandibular joint disorders are relatively common in the general population. Acute TMD symptoms such as pain, limitation of mandibular opening and impaired masticatory function are experienced in approximately 40% of the US population.[3] LeResche[4] reported that pain in the temporomandibular region occurs in 10% of the adult US population, involves mostly young and middle-aged adults, and has a female predilection. Another study reported that over a 6-month period, 10.8 million adults (6.0% of the US adult civilian population) experienced jaw joint and facial pain.[5] Women reported these symptoms 2.1 times more frequently than men. TMD symptoms have a peak occurrence between ages 20 and 40 years and are reported to be more prevalent in women than in men.[6] Studies show that approximately 5% of people with symptoms seek treatment.

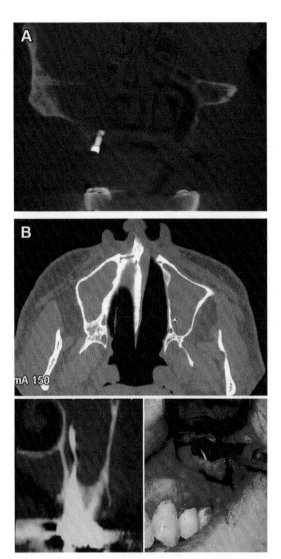

Fig. 3. (*A*) 60-year-old well-controlled diabetic patient with chronic congestion and discomfort of the right side of the face after dental implant placement. This cone beam scan demonstrates a completely opacified right maxillary sinus and an implant that has entered the maxillary sinus. Removal of the implant along with a Caldwell-Luc maxillary antrotomy and debridement revealed aspergillosis as the cause of the maxillary sinusitis. The removal of the pathology along with a 2-month course of antifungal medication resulted in complete resolution of the maxillary sinusitis. (*B*) Image of a 51-year-old man with onset of severe left-sided dental pain 2 days after endodontic therapy on a maxillary left first molar tooth. The diagnosis was acute maxillary sinusitis caused by reaction to endodontic material placed beyond the apex of the palatal root of the maxillary left first molar. Removal of the foreign body material, debridement, and evacuation of infected material from the maxillary sinus along with a course of antibiotics resulted in complete resolution of this infection.

Pathogenesis of Inflammatory/Degenerative Temporomandibular Joint Disorders

Internal derangement theory: a flawed approach to temporomandibular joint disorders

Internal derangement refers to a displaced position of the articular disk (usually anteriorly) of the temporomandibular joint. This condition was once considered to be central in the pathogenesis of temporomandibular joint disorders.[7] Anterior disk displacement was believed to be the major cause of intra-articular symptoms. The progression from anterior disk displacement to osteoarthritis and disk perforation was erroneously believed to be inevitable; therefore, conservative and surgical treatments were designed to reposition a displaced disk. Acceptance of the internal derangement theory led to flawed treatments without a valid research basis. As disk displacement is extremely common in asymptomatic individuals, our current understanding of temporomandibular joint pathogenesis does not support therapeutic interventions designed to reposition or replace a diseased disk.[8]

Current research has presented overwhelming evidence that temporomandibular joint disk displacement is the end result of changes in biochemistry and tissues caused by external factors such as overload and lack of movement. Ultimately, these external factors lead to tissue failure and altered joint biomechanics.

Patients with disk displacement presenting as a clicking joint, without significant symptoms of pain or altered range of motion, do not require surgical treatment. The clinician should view disk displacement as a flaw in joint biomechanics, which has occurred as a result of joint overloading. Disk displacement may be totally asymptomatic without any pain or limitation of function. Much research has been performed on temporomandibular joint pathology over the past 2 decades. The results of findings from clinical studies, magnetic resonance imaging (MRI) studies and synovial fluid analyses have provided compelling evidence that internal derangement theory as a major pathologic entity is flawed.[8–19] Research performed by Stegenga and colleagues[20,21] has furthered our understanding of temporomandibular joint pathogenesis, resulting in cartilage degradation. These studies concluded that abnormal disk position is the end result of degenerative changes that occur within the articular tissues.

Synovial fluid analysis research has provided great insight into the pathogenesis of inflammatory and degenerative conditions involving the temporomandibular joint. Studies involving obtaining synovial fluid samples and correlating the biochemical changes in the fluid with the morphologic alterations seen with arthroscopy have been extremely valuable. Biochemical changes and alteration in the structure and function of the synovial joint tissues occur in response to joint overloading and immobilization. Elevations in levels of inflammatory mediators[12,13,22] and proteoglycan degradation products[15,16,23,24] occur in the synovial fluids of pathologic temporomandibular joints. These biochemical abnormalities result in morphologic changes in the tissues including synovial inflammation and cartilage degradation (fibrillation). Osteoarthritis results in breakdown of the articular cartilage, which also impairs the sliding ability of opposing articular surfaces. Synovial inflammation causes pain and impaired lubrication leading to reduction in joint mobility. The combination of synovial inflammation and immobilization leads to temporomandibular joint adhesions, resulting in a further decrease in mobility.[25] Orthopedic studies[26,27] have shown that joint immobilization leads to adhesions, impaired cartilage nutrition, and cartilage degradation. Therefore, in patients with painful limitation of mandibular opening due to synovitis and osteoarthritis, there is a cycle of joint overloading leading to synovitis and osteoarthritis and reduced joint mobility. This condition leads to further adhesions, decreases in joint motion, pain, and more cartilage degradation (**Fig. 4**).

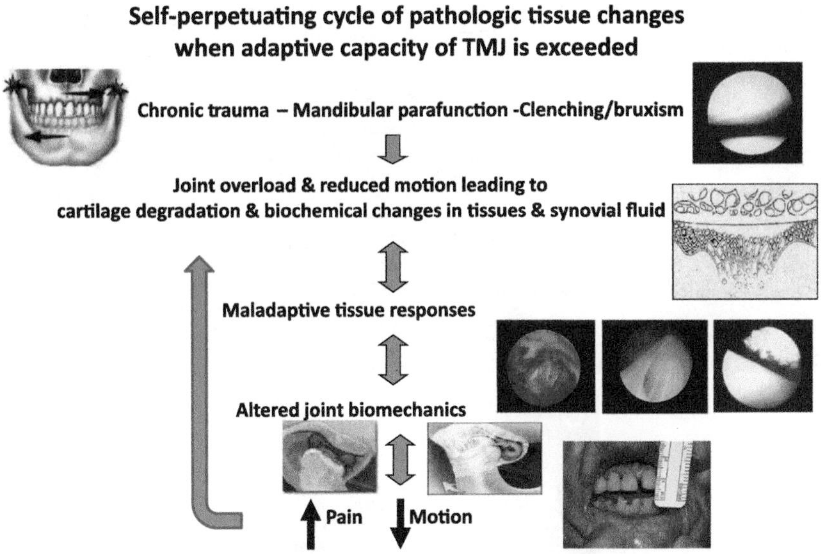

**Self-perpetuating cycle of pathologic tissue changes
when adaptive capacity of TMJ is exceeded**

Chronic trauma – Mandibular parafunction -Clenching/bruxism

⇩

Joint overload & reduced motion leading to
cartilage degradation & biochemical changes in tissues & synovial fluid

⇕

Maladaptive tissue responses

⇕

Altered joint biomechanics

⇕

↑ Pain   ↓ Motion

Fig. 4. Excessive loading of a synovial joint leads to biochemical alterations causing maladaptive tissue responses, including synovitis, osteoarthritis, and adhesions. Pathologic failure of these tissues lead to pain and altered mobility, which then lead to a cycle of further limitation of mobility, pain, and progression of tissue damage.

Maladaptive changes in synovial joints

Successful management of temporomandibular joint pathology must be based on reducing the external factors that lead to the underlying tissue abnormalities. The 2 major factors that contribute to the loss of structure and function of the temporomandibular joint are joint overloading and joint immobilization. Joint overloading, is usually caused by parafunctional masticatory habits such as clenching or bruxism. When excessive joint loading exceeds the adaptive capacity of the tissue, cartilage degradation occurs. Cartilage degradation products in the synovial fluid lead to synovitis.

Decreased joint mobility also leads to maladaptive tissue responses. Because movement is necessary for the diffusion of synovial fluid through cartilage to provide nutrition of chondrocytes, failure of this movement leads to chondrocyte death, leading to a failure of matrix production and a further breakdown of the articular cartilage. Reduced mobility, as well as the pain from synovial inflammation, leads to the formation of intra-articular adhesions, which further reduces mobility. These factors ultimately lead to a self-perpetuating cycle of reduced range of motion, synovitis, adhesions, and osteoarthritis (see **Fig. 4**).

Maladaptive changes in the tissues can be seen arthroscopically. Osteoarthritis (**Fig. 5**A), synovitis (see **Fig. 5**B), and adhesions (see **Fig. 5**C) are the major tissue pathologies that lead to altered joint biomechanics, pain, and limitation of function. These maladaptive tissue changes are not independent of each other and often coexist within the same damaged joint.

The clinical evaluation

A complete history and clinical examination are the most important diagnostic tools to establish a correct diagnosis. Having the patient point directly to the perceived location of the pain is extremely helpful. Pain due to intra-articular pathology is often well localized to the temporomandibular joint, tends to be more acute in nature, and is

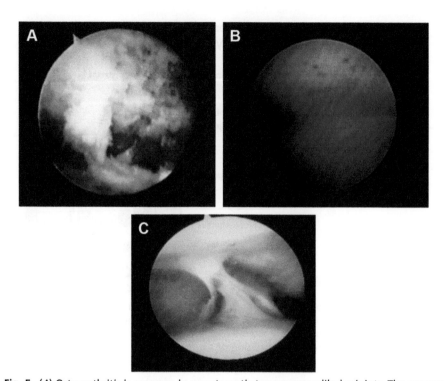

Fig. 5. (*A*) Osteoarthritis is common in symptomatic temporomandibular joints. The process of cartilage degradation because of joint overload leads to the appearance of fibrillation of the articular tissues. (*B*) Arthroscopic view of a temporomandibular joint with a grade 3 synovitis. The inflamed synovial tissues cause pain and swelling, leading to decreased joint movement and adhesions. The temporomandibular joint is constantly being loaded to permit the functions of eating, speaking, and swallowing. The presence of synovial inflammation and swelling along with further function and joint loading leads to further exacerbation and perpetuation of the inflammatory process. (*C*) Adhesions occur in the presence of continued synovitis and limited joint motion, which leads to a further decrease in mobility.

often associated with mandibular movement. Masticatory muscle pain is more diffuse in location and tends to be of a dull aching quality. The chronologic history should include when and how the symptoms began as well as assessment of past treatments and their effectiveness. A positive history of mandibular parafunction (clenching and bruxism) is an important finding. However, a negative history does not necessarily mean that there is an absence of the habit. Patients are often unaware of parafunctional habits, and they should be informed to become more aware of this habit.

Systemic conditions may manifest themselves in the temporomandibular joint and surrounding structures, creating symptoms that may initially seem to be due to local pathology. Therefore, a thorough medical history is required to determine if there are any systemic conditions, such as multiple sclerosis, rheumatoid arthritis, or other connective tissue disorders, that may be the cause of the symptoms.

The clinical examination should include the neck, extraoral structures, and intraoral structures. Examination of the dentition can reveal significant wear patterns on the occlusal surfaces of the teeth, providing secondary evidence of mandibular parafunction. Because the normal rest position of the mandible is with the teeth apart, a good clue to persistent clenching is to ask patients if they are aware of their upper and lower teeth touching during the day, when they are not eating. Once informed of this, patients often indicate that their teeth are together most of the day while they encounter the stresses of their daily life. The occlusion should also be evaluated; however, current research concerning an etiologic relationship between a malocclusion and TMD has failed to establish a definitive relationship.[28,29] An important symptom is an occlusion that is changing and getting worse. The patient often states that "my bite feels off and it is getting worse." Although tumors of the condyle and temporomandibular joint structures are not common, a progressive opening of the occlusion on one side is often the major symptom associated with a slowly expanding neoplasm in this region. An osteochondroma of the condyle is the most common tumor involving the temporomandibular joint (**Fig. 6**A–H).

The extraoral examination should include palpation of the temporomandibular joints including the lateral and posterior capsules (endaurally) to determine if there is tenderness. Pain due to palpation of the capsule is often a sign of synovial inflammation. Mandibular range of motion measurements should be obtained vertically as well as laterally. Maximum vertical opening is measured with a ruler from the incisal edge of the upper and lower central incisors (see **Fig. 1**, normal interincisal opening distance ranges from 35 to 55 mm). Deviation of the mandibular midline to one side during opening movements should be noted and usually represents a failure of translatory movement (sliding forward of the condyle along the articular eminence) on the side to which the mandible is deviating. Lateral excursion distances to the right and left are measured from the midline of the maxillary central incisor teeth to the midline of the mandibular central incisor teeth. Normal lateral excursions usually range from 8 to 15 mm and should not be painful. Protrusive (forward) mandibular movements should be performed, and any deviation should be noted.

Palpation of the muscles of mastication and the presence of tenderness is often a sign of myalgia or muscle spasm. The masseters, temporalis, as well as lateral and medial pterygoid muscles should be palpated bilaterally. Some patients have masseteric or temporalis hypertrophy, with extensive thickening of the muscles that can be seen simply by examining the face. Hypertrophied, firm, and enlarged muscles are usually signs of a mandibular parafunction.

Auscultation of the temporomandibular joints with a stethoscope should be performed to determine if there is clicking and/or crepitus. As TMJ sounds are common in the general population, the clinical significance of joint noise is questionable. Crepitus is often associated with degenerative joint conditions such as osteoarthritis. Clicking noises are associated with internal derangements (disk displacement) of the temporomandibular joint. Joint noise, in general, represents a biomechanical change in the joint as a response to joint overload.

The cranial nerve examination is an essential part of any thorough head and neck. For patients with chronic orofacial pain conditions, a thorough cranial nerve examination is essential and should be performed frequently at follow-up visits. When checking the facial nerve, it is important to determine if the weakness involves the entire side of the face or a portion of the face:

- A complete paralysis of one side of the face is usually an indication of a lower motor neuron lesion.
- If just the lower branches of the facial nerve are involved, this is more likely to be an upper motor neuron lesion.

The distinction between these 2 types of facial nerve dysfunction is important. The temporal branches of the facial nerve on one side receive input from upper motor

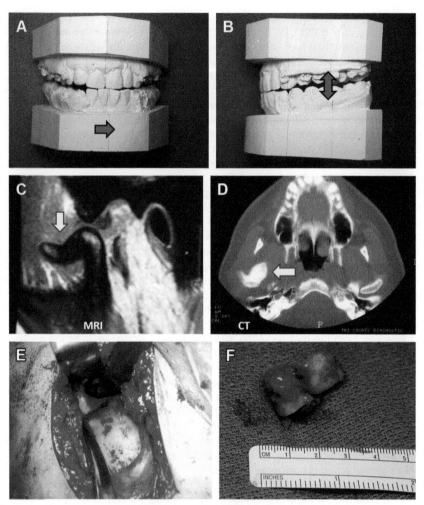

Fig. 6. (*A, B*) A 50-year-old woman presented with complaints of pain in the right temporomandibular joint and progressive shifting of her jaw to the left (*arrow*) causing an altered occlusion and facial asymmetry. The patient was treated for 2 years for a temporomandibular disorder with a night guard appliance; however, the symptoms progressed. Study models were obtained that demonstrated shifting of the mandible to the left and a posterior open bite (*arrows*). (*C, D*) MRI and computed tomography reveal a mass emanating from the right condyle (*arrows*). A tentative diagnosis of osteochondroma of the right mandibular condyle was made since this is the most common tumor involving the temporomandibular joint. (*E, F*) The osteochondroma was removed and an autogenous reconstruction was performed which restored the patient to a normal occlusion and total resolution of symptoms. (*G, H*) Postoperative radiograph following condylectomy and autogenous reconstruction resulting in a stable occlusion and correction of the facial asymmetry. The patient is currently 6 years postoperatively without any evidence of recurrence of the tumor or symptoms.

neurons bilaterally, because of decussation of these nerve fibers in the brain. The lower peripheral branches of the facial nerve receive upper motor neuron input from the ipsilateral side only. Thus, a centrally located lesion that affects the facial nerve will cause paralysis of only the lower half of the face. A peripherally located lesion

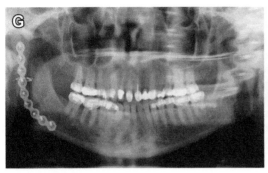
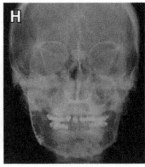

Fig. 6. (*continued*)

that affects the facial nerve, such as a parotid tumor, is likely to cause paralysis of all branches of the facial nerve on the side of the tumor.

Individuals who complain of sensory disturbances require a careful sensory examination. The simplest form of this examination is to map the area of altered sensation. A photograph will serve as a reference point to determine if the area of altered sensation is changing. If the map of the area of altered sensation follows the distribution of one of the sensory nerves, then it is highly suggestive of a pathologic condition or trauma that is altering normal sensory activity. Further investigation of both peripheral and central causes of altered sensory activity is required. Local pathology can often be diagnosed with radiographs and diagnostic images (computed tomography [CT] or MRI). Pathologic condition of the central nervous system that alters sensation requires an MRI and/or CT of the brain. Demyelinating diseases, such as multiple sclerosis, and intracranial tumors, such as acoustic neuroma, are common central causes of altered sensation involving the orofacial structures. Patients with masticatory muscle spasm often have intermittent areas of altered sensation that do not follow an anatomic distribution, which is most likely because of the effect of increased muscle activity causing intermittent impingement of terminal sensory fibers.

Radiographic evaluation of the maxilla, mandible, and temporomandibular joints is often necessary for completion of the examination. A panoramic radiograph is a tomogram of the maxilla and mandible and is nonspecific but useful as a screening tool for gross hard tissue pathology that may be present. The panoramic examination can reveal dental pathology, infections, maxillary sinusitis, facial fractures, and significant bony pathologies of the temporomandibular joint (**Fig. 7**). Bilateral temporomandibular

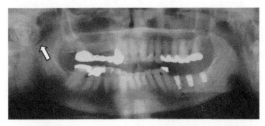

Fig. 7. An 80-year-old woman with no symptoms undergoes a routine panoramic radiographic examination for evaluation for implants. The panoramic radiograph demonstrates severe osteoarthritis of the right temporomandibular joint with heterotopic bone formation (*arrow*). No temporomandibular joint treatment is necessary because the patient is asymptomatic. This case demonstrates that diagnostic images do not necessarily correlate with the clinical examination or the presence of symptoms.

joint radiographs in the open and closed positions can be obtained from most panoramic equipment and are helpful in the assessment of temporomandibular joint structure and function. Panoramic radiographs are readily available in most oral and maxillofacial surgery offices. However, a limitation of the panoramic radiograph is that it will only demonstrate significant bony pathology, and therefore, it is not a sensitive technique for diagnosing intra-articular temporomandibular joint pathology. Cone beam scans are now readily available in many oral and maxillofacial surgery offices, which provide a low-cost, low-radiation option for obtaining a CT scan of the temporomandibular joints in the axial, coronal, and sagittal planes, as well as 3-dimensional reconstruction. A cone beam or CT scan of the temporomandibular joints is most useful for seeing bony pathology such as tumors, bony/fibrous ankylosis, and osteoarthritis (Fig. 8).

MRI has been extremely helpful in more recent years in the diagnosis of soft tissue pathology. Synovial joint effusion, osteoarthritis, and disk displacements can be detected with MRIs of the TMJ (Fig. 9). Recent studies have demonstrated a high incidence of disk displacement in asymptomatic subjects[9,30,31]; therefore, the clinician must use diagnostic imaging as an adjunct to the overall evaluation of the patient. Advanced diagnostic imaging should be performed when patients do not respond to conservative treatment or when there is clinical and radiographic evidence that significant pathologic condition, such as neoplasia, exists.

Principles of Nonsurgical Management of Inflammatory/Degenerative Temporomandibular Joint Disorders

The most common symptoms that are associated with temporomandibular joint disease are intra-articular pain, limitation of mandibular range of motion, and joint noises (clicking and/or crepitus). As these symptoms are nonspecific, they can reflect common temporomandibular joint pathologies, such as synovitis, adhesions, and osteoarthritis, or they may reflect more serious conditions such as neoplasia (osteochondroma and chondrosarcoma), fibrous/bony ankylosis, or systemic conditions (rheumatoid arthritis, psoriatic arthritis). The principles of treatment are also based on an accurate diagnosis

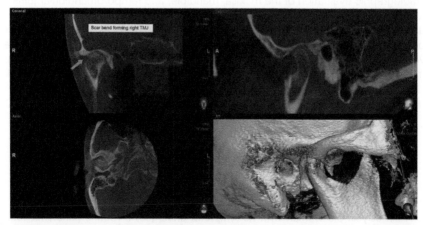

Fig. 8. Cone beam scan of the right temporomandibular joint in a patient with significant restriction in mandibular opening due to intra-articular pathology. The cone beam demonstrates early osteoarthritic changes as well as the development of scar tissue that is beginning to calcify (*arrow*). This patient has a fibrous ankylosis, which will lead to a bony ankylosis without further treatment.

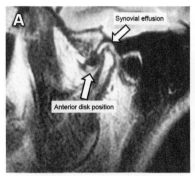
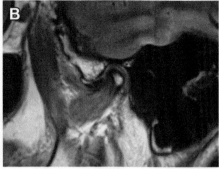

Fig. 9. (*A*) MRI T2 images demonstrating a significant synovial effusion and anterior disk position. (*B*) MRI demonstrating significant osteoarthritic changes. A disk perforation was present when the patient underwent arthroscopic surgery.

and a thorough understanding of the pathogenesis of the disease process. The following concepts are essential in the nonsurgical treatment of patients:

Reduction of joint loading

As joint overload leads to cartilage degradation, the clinician must be aware of parafunctional masticatory activities and control their deleterious effects. A soft nonchew diet for a specified period is necessary to reduce loading of the temporomandibular joint and associated muscles.

Patients' education involves informing them of the deleterious effects of clenching and making them aware of episodes in which their teeth come together during times of stress. Occlusal splint appliances are sometimes fabricated by the patient's dentist to distribute the forces equally between the maxillary and mandibular teeth during mandibular parafunction. These appliances work best in individuals with chronic pain from masticatory muscles. It is important to understand that these appliances do not prevent clenching and bruxism. The clinician must carefully evaluate the patient's response to these appliances because some individuals tend to clench more when there is an appliance in their mouth.

Maximize joint mobility

Orthopedic research has shown that joint immobilization has deleterious effects. Immobilization leads to joint adhesion and muscle atrophy. Passive motion exercises are an important part of synovial joint rehabilitation. Passive motion occurs when joint movement does not involve the use of the muscle groups that normally move the joint.

Passive motion exercises performed as a daily routine at home are essential for the restoration of normal joint mobility. Passive motion therapy for the temporomandibular joint can be achieved with a variety of devices designed to move the mandible by squeezing the device by hand (**Fig. 10**). Patients are generally instructed to perform these exercises for 5 minutes 3 to 4 times daily, after massage or moist heat applications. Frequent moist heat applications, massage, and ice applications are important adjuncts to passive motion exercises and help to reduce masticatory muscle spasm and myalgia. A great advantage of home passive motion exercises by patients is that their own proprioception can be used to achieve the maximum stretch without creating significant pain.

Reduction of inflammation and pain

If the patient attempts to function on inflamed synovial tissues, more inflammation is stimulated. For this reason, it is often quite difficult to reduce temporomandibular joint

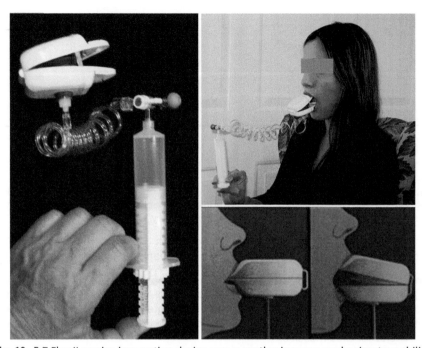

Fig. 10. E-Z Flex II passive jaw motion device uses a gentle air pump mechanism to mobilize the mandible. When the patient depresses the plunger, air from the syringe causes gentle separation of the upper and lower members of the mouthpiece. This device is used in patients with limitation of jaw opening from temporomandibular disorders as well as from other causes. Use of passive motion in patients undergoing radiation therapy to the head and neck for oral and pharyngeal cancer is necessary to prevent radiation-induced trismus. (*Courtesy of* Therapeutic Mobilization Devices, LLC, Great Neck, NY; with permission.)

inflammation as a result of constant use of the TMJ involved in speech, chewing, swallowing, and so on. However, inflammation of synovial tissues must be controlled for the temporomandibular joint to recover normal joint function. The inflammatory process can often be managed with nonsteroidal antiinflammatory medications, such as ibuprofen and naproxen. Unfortunately, it is common for patients to use these medications improperly by discontinuing use of the medication once the pain subsides in conjunction with attempts to resume a normal diet, causing reoccurrence of the symptoms because of persistent joint inflammation. For nonsteroidal antiinflammatory medications to be effective, they must be taken for at least 7 to 14 days, in conjunction with joint unloading, to attempt to reduce synovial inflammation. Some patients benefit from a short course of steroid medications; however, steroids should be used sparingly and generally reserved for acute exacerbations of synovial inflammation that are unresponsive to nonsteroidal antiinflammatory medications. If this course of treatment fails to significantly reduce the symptoms, it is an indication that the synovial inflammation is unlikely to be reversible with standard nonsurgical treatment.

Pain management is a necessary component of patient management. Failure to control pain levels, along with chronic tissue injury, has the potential to lead to central sensitization of ascending nerve pathways that transmit pain, leading to chronic neuropathic pain. This pain leads to symptoms of allodynia, in which nonnoxious stimuli, such as light touch, activate pain pathways leading to the cerebral cortex. An important goal in the management of these patients is to prevent the onset of chronic central neuropathic pain. With the onset of chronic neuropathic pain, local treatment of the diseased joint as well as a reduction in the activity of the central pain pathways is needed. However, successful management of the patient who has developed chronic neuropathic pain is much more difficult, because multiple surgical procedures and repeated trauma to tissues tend to exacerbate central sensitization of the ascending pain pathways.[32–38]

Local anesthetic injections to reduce pain may be helpful in the management of chronic neuropathic pain in conjunction with medications (anticonvulsants, such as gabapentin) that reduce activity of nerve pathways. Narcotic analgesics generally are not recommended in the management of chronic temporomandibular joint pain, because the pain relief is often brief, followed by rebound pain. A short course of narcotic analgesics can be prescribed for the management of postoperative pain. For patients who have complex chronic pain that does not respond to the aforementioned modalities, referral to a pain management specialist is recommended.

Recognize and treat masticatory muscle disorders
Masticatory muscle spasm is common in patients with COHFP, irrespective of the source of the pain, and represents a natural response to immobilize injured tissues. Patients who have severe pain from intra-articular temporomandibular joint pathology will often have significant masticatory muscle spasm and myalgia (muscle pain). Because joint overload from parafunctional masticatory activity is a common factor leading to joint pathology, it is often difficult for the clinician to determine whether the main pathology is intra-articular, with secondary masticatory muscle spasm, or it is masticatory muscle spasm and myalgia, with secondary joint inflammation. Muscle relaxant medications, massage, heat, and passive motion exercises are often helpful in treating chronic masticatory muscle spasm.

Relationship Between TMDs and Headache

Many patients with TMDs complain of headaches. The prevalence of headache in patients with TMD has been reported to be as high as 70% to 85%.[39–41] There is evidence that disorders of the masticatory muscles, related to parafunctional activities such as clenching or nocturnal bruxism, may be related to tension headache.[41–45] Because both headache and TMD symptoms are extremely common, the precise relationship between these 2 conditions is not known. A daily headache that occurs on awakening is often a symptom related to nocturnal bruxism. Patients frequently point to the temporalis muscle region as the primary location of their morning headache. Some patients indicate that stressful periods during the day cause them to clench their teeth and are associated with the symptoms of headache and diffuse jaw pain in the masseter and temporalis regions. If it has been determined that the cause of the headache is masticatory muscle spasm, and other causes of head pain have been ruled out, the treatment is the same as described previously for masticatory muscle disorders. However, it is important for the patient with headache to get a thorough neurologic evaluation to rule out other potential pathologic conditions. Referral to a neurologist and a brain MRI are often a necessary part of the workup.

Principles of Surgical Management of Temporomandibular Joint Disorders

Temporomandibular joint surgery is not a common treatment of routine temporomandibular joint disorders. However, when there is true intra-articular pathology and mandibular dysfunction that does not respond to routine treatment, surgical intervention is likely to be needed. The indications for performing temporomandibular joint surgery in the population of patients with significant temporomandibular joint symptoms and pathologic condition are as follows:

1. The patient has severe pain and/or mandibular dysfunction.
2. The cause of the pain and/or mandibular dysfunction is a diagnosis consistent with significant intra-articular pathology (usually synovitis, osteoarthritis, adhesions).
3. A full course of appropriate nonsurgical therapy has failed to improve the patient's symptoms.

Temporomandibular joint surgery does not necessarily reduce pain (unless if the sensory innervation to the joint is disrupted) but is designed to restore joint structure and function, and patients must understand that the postoperative period requires significant rehabilitation. With proper patient selection, appropriate surgery, and postoperative compliance with passive motion exercises, medications, and reduction of joint loads, most patients will ultimately have significant reduction in pain levels and improvement in mandibular functioning.

The principles of surgical management are as follows:

1. The least invasive procedure with the highest benefit to risk ratio should be performed.
2. Surgical procedures should be designed to remove and/or treat the pathologic tissue that is present.
3. Surgical procedures should assist in the reduction of synovial inflammation. Arthroscopic surgery enables the surgeon to isolate the areas of synovitis and inject a high concentration of antiinflammatory medication under direct vision into the most inflamed synovial tissues.
4. Surgical procedures should result in maximum preservation of the synovium, articular cartilage, and disk.
5. All operative procedures, whether performed under general anesthesia, conscious sedation, or local anesthesia, should be accompanied by the administration of local anesthesia to the surgical site. This administration will prevent barrages of noxious stimuli transmitted by peripheral sensory nerves from reaching the central nervous system.

The surgical options that are available to treat the more common temporomandibular joint disorders include arthrocentesis, arthroscopy, and arthrotomy. For patients who have a joint space, and have a clinical diagnosis of synovitis, osteoarthritis, and/or adhesions, arthrocentesis and arthroscopy are the least invasive surgical options. Arthrocentesis involves the insertion of 2 needles into the superior joint space and irrigating the joint with normal saline or lactated Ringer solution. Arthrocentesis is generally more effective when the onset of symptoms is of a relatively short duration, usually less than 3 months. Arthrocentesis is not effective if there are joint adhesions. Another disadvantage of arthrocentesis is that the actual pathologic condition cannot be visualized. A biopsy specimen cannot be obtained for histopathologic examination. Over recent years, temporomandibular joint arthroscopic surgery is being performed more frequently in an office setting.[46] Arthroscopic surgery has the advantage of permitting direct visualization and treatment of intra-articular pathology and when performed by an experienced surgeon, is minimally invasive. Thus, H.A.I. now rarely performs arthrocentesis because in office, arthroscopic surgery has significant advantages.

Arthroscopic temporomandibular joint surgery has the advantage of being minimally invasive, does not require incisions or sutures, and is associated with a rapid recovery, compared to open joint surgery. The procedure is performed in an ambulatory setting (either in the operating room or in a properly equipped office setting) permitting the patient to recover at home on the same day of the surgery. Once diagnostic arthroscopy has been completed, the areas of pathology can be identified. A second portal of entry enables the surgeon to perform operative procedures under direct vision with the arthroscope being present in one portal and the surgical instruments entering through the second portal. Operative arthroscopic surgery is designed to treat the pathologic condition that is present with maximum preservation of intra-articular tissues (**Fig. 11A–F**). Adhesions are released with miniblades and removed with alligator forceps or motorized shaving instruments. Synovitis is treated by directly isolating the most inflamed tissue and injection of a high concentration of steroid medication in the subsynovial tissues under direct vision. Identifying and treating synovial inflammation is an important part of this procedure. Osteoarthritic fibrillation tissue is removed with forceps and/or motorized shaving instruments. The removal of tissue specimens enables the surgeon to obtain histopathologic confirmation of the correct diagnosis. Occasionally, other uncommon pathologic conditions are diagnosed such as synovial chondromatosis, chondrocalcinosis, and pigmented villonodular synovitis. Anteriorly displaced disks are mobilized to improve translation in the superior joint space. Although there are some arthroscopic surgeons who stabilize the disk in a posterior position through a variety of techniques, H.A.I. opines that this is not necessary or indicated, because there are many asymptomatic individuals with anterior disk position.

Open joint surgery, which formerly was the mainstay of surgical treatment of the patient with intra-articular pathology, still has a place in the armamentarium of the oral and maxillofacial surgeon for the treatment of extensive intra-articular temporomandibular joint pathology. Because less-invasive procedures such as arthroscopy have a proven record of success in treating painful intra-articular pathologies, these modalities should be considered first. However, when the joint space is obliterated by fibrous and/or bony ankylosis, arthrotomy is the surgical treatment of choice. Conditions such as neoplasia (osteochondroma), synovial chondromatosis, and pigmented villonodular synovitis require open joint surgical procedures to remove the pathologic condition and restore joint function. There are numerous methods of reconstructing temporomandibular joints including autogenous reconstruction, distraction osteogenesis, and alloplastic temporomandibular joint reconstruction (**Fig. 12**).

The development of fibrous or bony ankylosis of the temporomandibular joint after arthroplasty is a potential risk of open joint surgery (**Fig. 13**). Because excellent outcomes can be achieved in these patients with a minimally invasive approach involving arthroscopic surgery, the authors believe that arthroplasty with disk repositioning surgery should be avoided.

Surgical outcomes

Studies reporting the outcomes of surgical treatment of temporomandibular joint disorders are usually retrospective cases series. These reports are fairly consistent, with reported success rates ranging from 75% to 90%.[47] Prospective, randomized, double-blind clinical studies are lacking and often impractical because most patients present with severe symptoms and a long history of failed nonsurgical treatments. Those patients who have been referred for a surgical evaluation are focused on treatments designed to relieve their symptoms, and these individuals are unlikely to submit to randomized treatments. Therefore, the published literature forces us to rely on reported case series to evaluate the outcomes of surgical treatment of temporomandibular joint disorders.

Numerous case studies on the outcomes of temporomandibular joint arthroscopy have demonstrated a significant reduction in pain, improved interincisal opening distance, and improved mandibular function without any change in disk position. Although

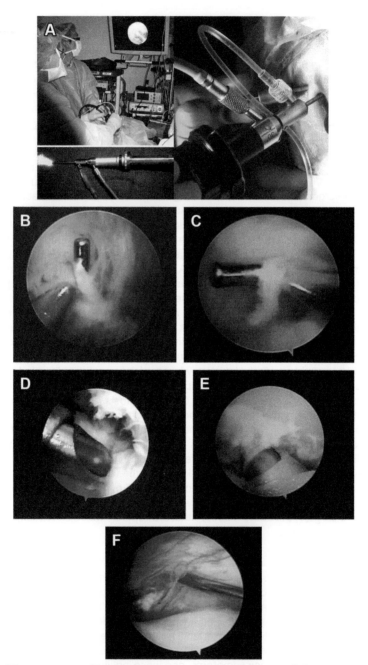

Fig. 11. (*A*) Temporomandibular joint arthroscopy setup. Because of the very small size of this joint, a very delicate arthroscope (usually 1.9 mm diameter or less) is used and special skills are needed by the surgeon to perform this operation successfully. (*B, C*) Operative arthroscopy demonstrating lysis of adhesions. (*D, E*) Operative arthroscopy with removal of pathologic osteoarthritic tissue with a motorized minishaver and a 2.0 full radius blade. (*F*) Direct injection of steroid (betamethasone 6 mg/mL) into areas of synovitis using a #25 gauge spinal needle.

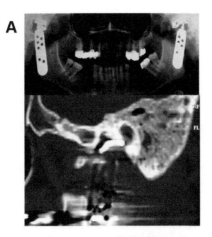

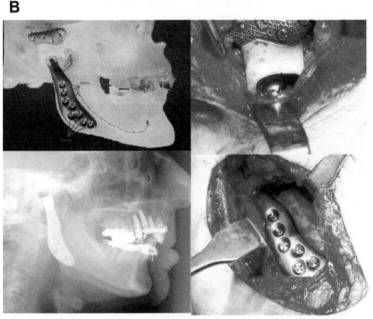

Fig. 12. (*A*) Failed alloplastic total joint reconstruction with poor materials and surgical technique from 15 years ago. This patient developed a chronic external otitis and mastoiditis because of erosion of the prosthesis into the external auditory canal. This older alloplastic total joint replacement system is no longer on the market. (*B*) Improved materials and surgical technique have resulted in successful alloplastic total joint replacement. This system (TMJ Concepts, Inc) is custom made on a 3-dimensional plastic model derived from a CT scan before surgical placement. A chrome cobalt condylar head articulates against ultrahigh molecular polyethylene fossa component. The fossa component is stabilized to the temporal bone with a custom-fitted titanium component and titanium screws. The mandibular condylar component is stabilized to the ramus of the mandible with a custom-fitted titanium component and titanium screws.

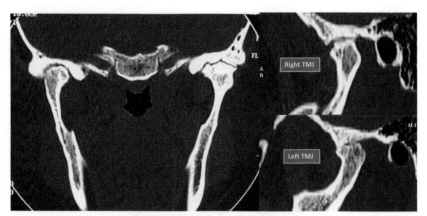

Fig. 13. Fibrous and bony ankylosis after multiple open temporomandibular joint surgeries including arthroplasty, followed by diskectomy. This patient needs chronic pain management and total joint replacement reconstruction.

ideal randomized controlled clinical studies evaluating the outcomes of arthroscopy do not exist, case series reports from different investigators have yielded remarkably consistent results. A compilation of 11 studies on the outcomes of arthroscopic surgery have demonstrated a mean success rate of 84%, with a mean reduction in pain levels on the visual analog scale of 4.6 after arthroscopy (mean follow-up 17.1 months) and a mean increase in interincisal opening distance of 10.4 mm.[48–58] These results are consistent with other published results on the outcomes of temporomandibular joint arthroscopy. A recent study compared the results of early versus late arthroscopic temporomandibular joint surgery.[59] Although both the early and late groups have significant reduction in pain and improvement in interincisal opening distance, the earlier group had better outcomes than the late group. This study suggests that prolonged unsuccessful nonsurgical therapy is not conservative and that early intervention with minimally invasive arthroscopic treatment can lead to improved outcomes.

Postoperative rehabilitation

Surgical procedures on the temporomandibular joint that are not followed by an appropriate postoperative rehabilitation regimen are very likely to fail. The surgeon must emphasize to the patient that the postoperative rehabilitation period is crucial in determining the outcome of the surgery. Postoperative rehabilitation designed to restore mandibular range of motion, prevent the formation of adhesions, reduce inflammation, and reduce the etiologic factors such as joint overloading are essential for surgical success.

Conceptually, the first goal after the surgery is to restore a normal mandibular range of motion. However, joint loading (chewing, mandibular parafunction) must be avoided. Although the regimen for each patient is different, based on their postoperative clinical course, the following are the general guidelines that are used. The patient is placed on a nonchew diet for approximately 3 weeks, to prevent loading of intraarticular tissues. This joint unloading is necessary to permit the tissues to recover, because early function and joint overload will precipitate the same factors that caused the initial pathologic condition. If the patient is minimally symptomatic by postoperative week 3, a gradual progression of the diet is permitted, as long as there is no exacerbation of pain or dysfunction. If pain occurs during chewing, the patient is instructed to continue on the nonchew diet for an additional week, until the loads of mastication on the temporomandibular joint are tolerated. If there is no pain during chewing, but if there is soreness in the muscles of mastication after chewing, this is to be expected due to disuse atrophy. Muscle atrophy from a prolonged period of mandibular dysfunction is present postoperatively, and a gradual return to function ultimately builds up the lost muscle strength.

Passive motion exercises are essential in the postoperative period and are necessary to prevent the formation of new adhesions and increase mandibular range of motion. A variety of techniques and devices are available to achieve passive range of motion exercises. H.A.I. prefers the use of E-Z Flex II (H.A.I. is the owner of TMD, LLC, Great Neck, New York, the manufacturer of E-Z Flex II), which uses an air pump mechanism that is gentle and promotes patient compliance (see **Fig. 10**). Other options for passive mandibular motion include other handheld devices, tongue blades, and finger stretching techniques. These exercises are performed thrice daily for 5 to 10 minutes, preceded by moist heat or massage, and followed by ice or massage. Physical therapy may be prescribed, particularly if the patient tends to be noncompliant with the exercises or if the patient's interincisal opening distance is not increasing as expected.

Postoperative pain management usually requires only a few days of narcotic analgesics. Long-term use of narcotics beyond the first postoperative week should be avoided. Nonsteroidal antiinflammatory medications and muscle relaxants (bedtime only) are frequently prescribed. Patients can usually return to their normal activities (work or school) within 4 to 7 days. Once the patient has an adequate range of mandibular motion and reduced pain (usually 4–12 weeks), the passive motion exercises are gradually reduced to twice daily, the consistency of the diet is advanced, and the medications are used as needed. Throughout the postoperative period, avoidance of those factors, such as mandibular parafunction, that contributed to the development of the temporomandibular joint disorder is essential. It is not uncommon for the patient with a high stress lifestyle to do quite well for a period while they are recuperating from the surgery. However, when patients return to their routine daily activities and the same demands and stresses at work or at home are placed on them, mandibular clenching habits return. It is important for the patient to become acutely aware of mandibular parafunction particularly during the day and to develop strategies for recognition and avoidance of habits that cause joint overload.

OTHER DISORDERS AFFECTING THE TEMPOROMANDIBULAR JOINT OF SPECIAL INTEREST TO THE OTOLARYNGOLOGIST
Radiation Fibrosis

Patients with oral and pharyngeal cancers who undergo radiation therapy require special consideration with respect to the importance of maintaining an adequate range of mandibular motion. It is well known that these patients are prone to recurrent cancers or new primary lesions. Thus, maintaining an acceptable interincisal opening distance is necessary to detect recurrent or second primary cancerous lesions at an early stage. Unfortunately, radiation therapy often causes fibrosis of the soft tissues including the muscles of mastication and the temporomandibular joint, resulting in severe restriction in mouth opening. Therefore, it is essential for these patients to perform passive motion exercises on a regular basis before, during, and after radiation therapy (see **Fig. 10**). The goal is to maintain and maximize mandibular range of motion to help offset the effects of radiation fibrosis causing trismus. Once radiation fibrosis and trismus has occurred, it is extremely difficult, if not impossible, to restore mandibular range of motion to an acceptable level. The importance of passive motion mandibular exercises to prevent trismus in patients before radiation therapy is often overlooked. Such overlooking is unfortunate because passive motion therapy is a simple, noninvasive therapy that can prevent or reduce trismus, ultimately improving quality of life and potentially permitting the early detection of oral and pharyngeal cancer.

The Relationship Between Tinnitus and TMDs

The association of tinnitus and other otologic symptoms with TMDs has been controversial, because Costen's article in 1934 reported direct causal relationships between temporomandibular joint disorders and tinnitus/otologia.[1] Objective tinnitus is caused by sounds generated in the body that reach the ear through conduction in body tissue. Subjective tinnitus is much more common, occurs without any physical sound reaching the ear, and is associated with abnormal neural activity generated in the ear, the auditory nerve, or the central nervous system.[60] Subjective tinnitus may occur with hearing loss after exposure to loud noise, after administration of certain drugs, as a symptom of vestibular schwannoma, or as a symptom of Meniere disease. However, most often the cause of tinnitus remains unknown.[60]

Epidemiologic studies have demonstrated tinnitus to be a common symptom in the general population, but with a higher prevalence in patients with TMD symptoms. One study reported the incidence of tinnitus to be 10% to 31% of the general population and up to 85% in the population of patients with TMD symptoms.[61] Another study reported similar findings, with 2 control populations having tinnitus in 13.8% and 32.5%, compared to a 59.6% prevalence of tinnitus in a population of patients with TMD symptoms.[62] The pathophysiological mechanisms between TMD and tinnitus are not well understood, and several attempts have been made to explain the associations.[62–64]

Morphologic and anatomic studies have confirmed a relationship between the middle ear and the temporomandibular joint through the connection between the malleus and the posterior capsule of the joint via the discomalleolar ligament.[65] The structures of the middle ear and TMJ are derived from the first brachial arch (mandibular arch) and thus are anatomically and morphogenically related. The discomalleolar ligament is an intrinsic fibrous ligament that connects the TMJ disk with the malleus of the middle ear. The discomalleolar ligament has fibers that attach to the upper lamina of the bilaminar zone of the articular disk of the temporomandibular joint. These fibers from the discomalleolar ligament attach to the posterosuperior and medial end of the articular disk and enter the middle ear through the most lateral portion of the petrotympanic fissure and the malleolar sulcus, ultimately attaching to the malleus.

The middle ear cavity is connected to the nasopharynx via the eustachian tube. Conditions that impair the opening of the eustachian tube can lead to the sensation of fullness or stuffiness in the ear.[66] Patients can somatically modulate tinnitus with jaw movements, swallowing, and external pressure on the temporomandibular joint.[67–69] The tensor tympani and tensor veli palatini are muscles that are necessary for normal eustachian tube function and are innervated by motor branches of the fifth cranial nerve. The muscles of mastication (masseter, temporalis, as well as medial and lateral pterygoids) are also innervated by the motor division of the fifth cranial nerve. In addition, noxious stimuli that affect the sensory branches of the fifth cranial nerve can affect ear sensations and cause a variety of otologic symptoms. Neural inputs of the trigeminal system are linked to the inner ear via the dorsal cochlear nucleus; thus, the central excitatory effects with the flexing and tightening on the tympanic membrane can bring about sensations of tinnitus and vertigo.[60,67,69] In spite of the close anatomic relationships between the temporomandibular joint, middle ear, eustachian tube, muscles of mastication, muscles of the nasopharynx, and the fifth cranial nerve, the precise mechanisms that produce the symptom of tinnitus remain to be elucidated.

Consistent with Costen's hypothesis are recent reports demonstrating that treatment of TMD symptoms often result in improvement of tinnitus and other otologic symptoms. In a study, 202 patients with TMD with coexisting tinnitus, otalgia, dizziness, and/or vertigo were treated for their TMD symptoms.[70] After satisfactory TMD symptom improvement was obtained, the percentage of subjects reporting significant improvement or resolution of their otologic symptoms was reported as follows: tinnitus 83%, otalgia 94%, dizziness 91%, and vertigo 100%. Other reports have suggested that otologic symptoms and tinnitus may improve with TMD therapy.[64,71–73] Methodological weaknesses of many of these studies have led others to conclude that the lack of prospective, controlled, and randomized studies regarding the effectiveness of TMD treatment as treatment of otalgia and tinnitus in patients with TMD are not well supported.[74] The influence of the placebo effect on otologic symptoms once TMD therapy is instituted cannot be overlooked. In spite of the uncertainty concerning the causal relationship between TMD therapy and otologic symptoms, it is important for the practicing clinician to provide the patient with an appropriate course of management. Therefore, if the patient has otologic symptoms that cannot be explained and if the otolaryngologist suspects the presence of a TMD, it is reasonable for the patient to be referred to a clinician with expertise in the diagnosis and management of TMDs and COHFP. If the consultation confirms the presence of a TMD, treatment of this disorder is certainly appropriate with an ongoing evaluation of the patient's signs and symptoms. If the otologic symptoms resolve, then one may conclude that there was perhaps a relationship between the TMD treatment and the otologic symptoms, although the placebo effect cannot be ruled out. If otologic symptoms persist, it is very important for the diagnosis and management to continue to be reevaluated with further intense workup for the correct diagnosis and course of treatment.

SUMMARY: THE ESSENTIAL ROLE OF THE OTOLARYNGOLOGIST IN DIAGNOSIS AND MANAGEMENT OF TEMPOROMANDIBULAR JOINT AND COHFP DISORDERS: A TEAM APPROACH

The specialist in otolaryngology is a key member of the team of physicians that diagnose and treat COHFP. Otalgia, headache, and facial pain are common symptoms in patients seeking consultation with the otolaryngologist. The challenge for each clinician is to be able to make an accurate diagnosis leading to appropriate timely treatment. Some patients have symptoms, signs, and clinical findings that are specific for local pathology, making diagnosis and treatment relatively clear and straightforward. Patients with COHFP as well as TMDs often have complex histories and clinical findings making it difficult to make an accurate diagnosis. The clinician must constantly reevaluate the patient's response to treatment to help confirm or negate the proposed diagnosis and to adjust treatment regimens accordingly.

When the diagnosis is unclear, referrals to appropriate specialists are a necessary component in the management of the patient with COHFP. Listed below are those specialties that are likely to be included in the management of the patient with chronic orofacial pain:

- Otolaryngology
- Oral and maxillofacial surgery
- Neurology
- Neurosurgery
- Rheumatology

- Psychiatry
- Psychology
- Anesthesiology
- General dentistry
- Endodontics
- Radiology
- Physical therapy
- Alternative medicine

The otolaryngologist should have a relationship with a group of specialists who are available to provide assistance in the diagnosis and management of the patient with COHFP. The clinician must be confident that these specialists are individuals who have the time, expertise, and willingness to take on the challenge of caring for these complex patients.

REFERENCES

1. Costen JB. A syndrome of ear and sinus symptoms dependent upon disturbed function of the temporomandibular joint. Ann Otol Rhinol Laryngol 1934;43(1): 1–15.
2. Kreiner M, Okeson JP, Michelis V, et al. Craniofacial pain as the sole symptom of cardiac ischemia: a prospective multicenter study. J Am Dent Assoc 2007; 138(1):74–9.
3. Scrivani SJ, Keith DA, Kaban LB. Temporomandibular disorders. N Engl J Med 2008;359:2693–705.
4. LeResche L. Epidemiology of temporomandibular disorders: implications for the investigation of etiologic factors. Crit Rev Oral Biol Med 1997;8(3): 291–305.
5. Lipton JA, Ship JA, Larach-Robinson D. Estimated prevalence and distribution of reported orofacial pain in the United States. J Am Dent Assoc 1993;124: 115–21.
6. Liu F, Steinkeler A. Epidemiology, diagnosis, and treatment of temporomandibular disorders. Dent Clin North Am 2013;57(3):465–79.
7. McCarty WL, Farrar WB. Surgery for internal derangements of the temporomandibular joint. J Prosthet Dent 1979;42(2):191–6.
8. Dolwick MF. Intra-articular disc displacement part I: its questionable role in temporomandibular joint pathology. J Oral Maxillofac Surg 1995;53:1069–72.
9. Moore JB. Coronal and sagittal TMJ meniscus position in asymptomatic subjects by MRI [abstract]. J Oral Maxillofac Surg 1989;47:75.
10. Kircos LT, Ortendahl DA, Mark AS, et al. Magnetic resonance imaging of the TMJ disc in asymptomatic volunteers. J Oral Maxillofac Surg 1987;45:852–4.
11. Trumpy IG, Lyberg T. Surgical treatment of internal derangement of the temporomandibular joint: long-term evaluation of three techniques. J Oral Maxillofac Surg 1995;53:746–7.
12. Quinn JH, Bazan NG. Identification of prostaglandin E2 and leukotriene B4 in the synovial fluid of painful, dysfunctional temporomandibular joints. J Oral Maxillofac Surg 1990;48:968.
13. Shafer DM, Assael L, White LB, et al. Tumor necrosis factor alpha as a biochemical marker of pain and outcome in temporomandibular joints with internal derangements. J Oral Maxillofac Surg 1994;52:786.
14. Kopp S. Neuroendocrine, immune and local responses related to temporomandibular disorders. J Orofac Pain 2001;15:9.

15. Ratcliffe A, Israel HA. Proteoglycan components of articular cartilage in synovial fluids as potential markers of osteoarthritis of the temporomandibular joint. In: Sessle BJ, Bryant PS, Dionne RA, editors. Temporomandibular disorders and related pain conditions, progress in pain research and management, vol. 4. Seattle (WA): IASP Press; 1995. p. 141–50.
16. Israel H, Diamond B, Saed-Nejad F, et al. Correlation between arthroscopic diagnosis of osteoarthritis and synovitis of the human temporomandibular joint and keratan sulfate levels in the synovial fluid. J Oral Maxillofac Surg 1997;55:210.
17. Kubota E, Imamura H, Kubota T, et al. Interleukin 1 beta and stromelysin (MMP3) activity of synovial fluid as possible markers of osteoarthritis in the temporomandibular joint. J Oral Maxillofac Surg 1997;55:20.
18. Kubota E, Kubota T, Matsumoto J, et al. Synovial fluid cytokines and proteinases as markers of temporomandibular joint disease. J Oral Maxillofac Surg 1998;56:192.
19. Israel H, Diamond B, Saed-Nejad F, et al. Osteoarthritis and synovitis as major pathoses of the temporomandibular joint: comparison of clinical diagnosis and arthroscopic morphology. J Oral Maxillofac Surg 1998;56:1023–8.
20. Stegenga B, DeBont LG, Boering G. Osteoarthrosis as the cause of craniomandibular pain and dysfunction: a unifying concept. J Oral Maxillofac Surg 1989; 47:249–56.
21. Stegenga B, DeBont LG, Boering G, et al. Tissue responses to degenerative changes in the temporomandibular joint: a review. J Oral Maxillofac Surg 1991;49:1079–88.
22. Chang H, Israel H. Analysis of inflammatory mediators in TMJ synovial fluid lavage samples in symptomatic patients and asymptomatic controls. J Oral Maxillofac Surg 2005;63:761–5.
23. Shibata T, Murakami KI, Kubota E, et al. Glycosaminoglycan components in temporomandibular joint synovial fluid as markers of joint pathology. J Oral Maxillofac Surg 1998;56:209.
24. Israel H, Saed-Nejad F, Ratcliffe A. Early diagnosis of osteoarthrosis of the temporomandibular joint: correlation between arthroscopic diagnosis and keratan sulfate levels in the synovial fluid. J Oral Maxillofac Surg 1991;49:708–11.
25. Israel H, Langevin CJ, Singer M. The relationship between temporomandibular joint synovitis and adhesions: pathogenic mechanisms and clinical implications for surgical management. J Oral Maxillofac Surg 2006;64:1066–74.
26. Salter RB. The biologic concept of continuous passive motion of synovial joints. The first 18 years of basic research and is clinical application. Clin Orthop 1989;242:12.
27. Akeson WH, Amiel D, Ing D, et al. Effects of immobilization on joints. Clin Orthop 1987;219:28.
28. National Institutes of Health Technology Assessment Conference Statement: management of temporomandibular disorders. J Am Dent Assoc 1996;127:1595–606.
29. Stohler C. Management of the dental occlusion. In: Laskin D, Greene C, Hylander W, editors. Temporomandibular disorders: an evidence-based approach to diagnosis and treatment. Chicago: Quintessence Publishing Company, Inc; 2006. p. 403–11.
30. Kircos LT, Douglas A, Mark AS, et al. Magnetic resonance imaging of the TMJ disc in asymptomatic volunteers. J Oral Maxillofac Surg 1987;45:852.
31. Katzberg RW, Westesson P, Tallents RH, et al. Anatomic disorders of the temporomandibular joint disc in asymptomatic subjects. J Oral Maxillofac Surg 1996; 54:147–53.
32. Robinson PP, Boissonade FM, Loescher AR, et al. Peripheral mechanisms for the initiation of pain following trigeminal nerve injury. J Orofac Pain 2004;18(4):287–92.

33. Dubner R, Ren K. Brainstem mechanisms of persistent pain following injury. J Orofac Pain 2004;18(4):299–305.
34. Salter M. Cellular neuroplasticity mechanisms mediating pain persistence. J Orofac Pain 2004;18(4):318–24.
35. Truelove E. Management issues of neuropathic trigeminal pain from a dental perspective. J Orofac Pain 2004;18(4):374–80.
36. Benoliel R, Eliav E, Elishoov H, et al. Diagnosis and treatment of persistent pain after trauma to the head and neck. J Oral Maxillofac Surg 1994;52(11):1138–47.
37. Israel H, Ward JD, Horrell B, et al. Oral and maxillofacial surgery in patients with chronic orofacial pain. J Oral Maxillofac Surg 2003;61:662–7.
38. Milam SB. Failed implants and multiple operations. Oral Surg Oral Med Oral Pathol Oral Radiol Endod 1997;83:156.
39. Magnusson T, Carlsson GE. Comparison between two groups of patients in respect to headache and mandibular dysfunction. Swed Dent J 1978;2:85–7.
40. Andrasik F, Holyroyd KA, Abell T. Prevalence of headache within a college student population: a preliminary analysis. Headache 1979;19:384–7.
41. Jensen R, Olesen J. Oromandibular dysfunction, tension type-headache, cluster headache and miscellaneous headaches. In: Olesen J, Tfelt-Hansen P, Welch KM, editors. The headache. New York: Raven; 1993. p. 479–82.
42. Forssell H, Kangasniemi P. Mandibular dysfunction in patients with muscle contraction headache. Proc Finn Dent Soc 1984;80:211–6.
43. Gelb H, Tarte J. A two year clinical dental evaluation of 200 cases of chronic headache: the cranio-cervical-mandibular syndrome. J Am Dent Assoc 1975;91:1230–6.
44. Heloe B, Heloe LA, Heiberg A. Relationship between sociomedical factors and TMJ symptoms in Norwegians with myofascial pain-dysfunction syndrome. Community Dent Oral Epidemiol 1977;5:207–12.
45. Jensen R, Rasmussen BK, Pedersen B, et al. Muscle tenderness and pressure pain thresholds in headache. A population study. Pain 1993;52:193–9.
46. Israel H, Lee A, Shum J, et al. Temporomandibular Joint Arthroscopy in the operating room versus office: is there a difference in outcomes? [abstract]. J Oral Maxillofac Surg 2010;68(Suppl 9):55–6.
47. Laskin D. Surgical management of internal derangements. In: Laskin D, Greene C, Hylander W, editors. An evidence-based approach to diagnosis and treatment. Chicago: Quintessence Publishing Company, Inc; 2006. p. 469–81.
48. Fridrich KL, Wise JM, Zeitler DL. Prospective comparison of arthroscopy and arthrocentesis for temporomandibular joint disorders. J Oral Maxillofac Surg 1996; 54:816.
49. Sanders B, Buoncristiani R. Diagnostic and surgical arthroscopy of the temporomandibular joint: clinical experience with 136 procedures over a 2-year period. J Craniomandib Disord 1987;1:202.
50. Moses JJ, Poker ID. TMJ arthroscopic surgery: an analysis of 237 patients. J Oral Maxillofac Surg 1989;47:790.
51. Indresano AT. Arthroscopic surgery of the temporomandibular joint: report of 64 patients with long-term follow-up. J Oral Maxillofac Surg 1989;47:439.
52. Israel H, Roser SM. Patient response to temporomandibular joint arthroscopy: preliminary findings in 24 patients. J Oral Maxillofac Surg 1989;47:570.
53. Montgomery MT, Van Sickels J, Harms SE, et al. Arthroscopic TMJ surgery: effects on signs, symptoms and disc position. J Oral Maxillofac Surg 1989;47:1263.
54. McCain JP, Sanders B, Koslin M, et al. Temporomandibular joint arthroscopy: a 6-year multicenter retrospective study of 4,831 joints. J Oral Maxillofac Surg 1992;50:926.

55. Hoffman DC, Cubillos L. The effect of arthroscopic surgery on mandibular range of motion. Cranio 1994;12(1):11.
56. Murakami K, Hosaka H, Moriya Y, et al. Short-term outcome study for the management of temporomandibular joint closed lock. Oral Surg Oral Med Oral Pathol 1995;80:253.
57. Murakami K, Moriya Y, Goto K, et al. Four-year follow-up study of temporomandibular joint arthroscopic surgery for advanced internal derangements. J Oral Maxillofac Surg 1996;54:285.
58. Chossegros C, Cheynet F, Gola R, et al. Clinical results of therapeutic temporomandibular joint arthroscopy: a prospective study of 34 arthroscopies with prediscal section and retrodiscal coagulation. Br J Oral Maxillofac Surg 1996; 34:504.
59. Israel H, Behrman D, Friedman J, et al. Early versus late intervention with arthroscopy for treatment of inflammatory temporomandibular joint disorders. J Oral Maxillofac Surg 2010;68(11):2661–7.
60. Moller AR. Tinnitus: presence and future. Prog Brain Res 2007;166:3–16.
61. Salvetti G, Manfredini D, Barsotti S, et al. Otologic symptoms in temporomandibular disorders patients: is there evidence of an association-relationship. Minerva Stomatol 2006;55(11–12):627–37.
62. Parker WS, Chole RA. Tinnitus, vertigo, and temporomandibular disorders. Am J Orthod Dentofacial Orthop 1995;107(2):153–8.
63. Chole RA, Parker WS. Tinnitus in patients with temporomandibular disorders. Arch Otolaryngol Head Neck Surg 1992;118(8):817–21.
64. Wright EF, Syms CA III, Bifano SL. Tinnitus, dizziness, and non-otologicotalgia improvement through temporomandibular disorder therapy. Mil Med 2000; 165(10):733–6.
65. Rodriguez-Vazquez JF, Merida-Velasco JR, Merida-Velasco JA, et al. Anatomical considerations on the discomalleolar ligament. J Anat 1998;192(4):617–21.
66. Okeson JP. Management of temporomandibular disorders and occlusion. 6th edition. Lexington (KY): Mosby; 2008. p. 164–204.
67. Levine RA, Abel M, Cheng H. CNS somatosensory-auditory interactions elicit or modulate tinnitus. Exp Brain Res 2003;153(4):643–8.
68. Lam DK, Lawrence HP, Tenenbaum HC. Aural symptoms in temporomandibular disorder patients attending a craniofacial pain unit. J Orofac Pain 2001;152(2): 146–57.
69. Shore S, Zhou J, Koehler S. Neural mechanisms underlying somatic tinnitus. Prog Brain Res 2007;166:107–23.
70. Wright EF. Otologic symptom improvement through TMD therapy. Quintessence Int 2007;38(9):564–71.
71. Tullberg M, Ernberg M. Long-term effect on tinnitus by treatment of temporomandibular disorders: a two-year follow-up by questionnaire. Acta Odontol Scand 2006;64(2):89–96.
72. Seedorf H, Leuwer R, Fenske C, et al. The "Costen Syndrome" - which symptoms suggest that the patient may benefit from dental therapy? Laryngorhinootologie 2002;81(4):268–75.
73. deFelicio CM, Melchior Mde O, Ferreira CL, et al. Otologic symptoms of temporomandibular disorders and effect of orofacial myofunctional therapy. Cranio 2008;26(2):118–25.
74. Turp JC. Correlation between myoarthropathies of the masticatory system and ear symptoms (otalgia, tinnitus). HNO 1998;46(4):303–10.

Vertiginous Headache and Its Management

Sujana S. Chandrasekhar, MD[a,b,c,d,*]

KEYWORDS

- Headache • Migraine • Dizziness • Vertigo • Meniere syndrome
- Ocular movement disorder

KEY POINTS

- Vertiginous headache may occur with the headache and the dizziness symptoms may occur simultaneously or at seemingly unrelated times.
- Patients may have a personal or family history of migraine headaches, with or without aura, and their symptoms are often described as atypical Meniere syndrome.
- Patients with vertiginous headache are often intolerant to complex visual stimuli, such as busy market aisles, action or 3-D movies, and scrolling on the computer, and motion sickness is a frequent finding.
- Evaluation for Meniere syndrome, migraine headache, and ocular vergence abnormalities is helpful in patients with vertiginous headache.
- Treatment is directed toward the underlying problem and may include migraine medication, Meniere treatment, and/or vision therapy directed to vergence stability.

OVERVIEW

Headache and dizziness are vague words used to describe symptoms that can encompass a range of discomfort experiences, from mild head pressure to severe, debilitating head pain, and from light-headedness or heavy-headedness to feeling off-balance or experiencing true spinning vertigo. As learned from the time of Osler,[1] careful, prompted history enables a patient help the physician determine the actual symptoms that the patient is experiencing and start to determine causality. The historical features of interest include duration of headache history, presence of vertigo or dizziness, frequency and length of headache or dizziness episodes, association of vertigo with either headache or the triggers or precipitants of the headache, aura, accompanying symptoms, and alleviating factors.[2–5] Personal or family history of headache

Disclosures: There are no pertinent disclosures.
[a] New York Otology, 1421 Third Avenue, 4th Floor, New York, NY 10028, USA; [b] James J. Peters Veterans Administration Medical Center, Bronx, NY, USA; [c] New York Head & Neck Institute, Northshore-LIJ Medical Center, New York, NY, USA; [d] Mount Sinai School of Medicine, New York, NY, USA
* New York Otology, 1421 Third Avenue, 4th Floor, New York, NY 10028.
E-mail address: ssc@nyotology.com

Otolaryngol Clin N Am 47 (2014) 333–341
http://dx.doi.org/10.1016/j.otc.2013.11.001
0030-6665/14/$ – see front matter © 2014 Elsevier Inc. All rights reserved.

or migraine, use of medications, and social history, including ingestion of caffeine, nicotine, and salt, are important. There is evidence that vertigo in childhood is associated with migraine headaches in adulthood.[6,7]

Migraine-Associated Vertigo

Approximately 13% of the adult population has migraine; of those, 27% to 42% report episodic vertigo, with more than one-third of them describing their vertigo as occurring during headache-free periods. These patients are also refractory to traditional vestibular rehabilitation and have been recently classified as having migraine-associated dizziness (MAD) or migraine-associated vertigo (MAV).[8] Criteria for diagnosis of MAD are evolving, but frequently patients with episodic dizziness or vertigo have only a remote history of migraine headache or vice versa. Often, these patients report episodic dizziness and/or headache brought on by complex visual stimuli.[9] Work-up can sometimes show unilateral vestibular hypofunction or abnormality on electrocochleography or vestibular evoked myogenic potential (VEMP) but often is normal. MRI often reveals findings, such as nonspecific white matter lesions, that are consistent with migraine. These dizzy patients who complain of intolerance to complex visual motion and who demonstrate normal vestibular function often fall into the category of MAD. A subset of these patients responds to migraine pharmacotherapy. Neuro-optometric examination of such patients frequently reveals a weakness of vergence ocular motility. In those patients, completion of a course of vision rehabilitation treatment (VT) can improve both symptoms and overall function.

Although the International Headache Society only recognizes vertigo as a component of basilar-type migraine,[10] many studies have sought to better define the relationship between migraine and vertigo. A prospective study examining 200 patients from a dizziness clinic and 200 patients from a migraine clinic were compared with 200 age-matched and gender-matched controls from an orthopedic clinic.[8] A statistically significant increase in the prevalence of migraine was demonstrated in the dizziness clinic group (38%) versus the orthopedic control group (24%). In contrast to visual vertigo patients, however, vestibular function tests, including caloric testing and dynamic posturography, often fail to demonstrate a vestibular weakness in MAV patients.[11]

Motion Sickness

A lower threshold for motion sickness susceptibility has been shown in migraine patients. One study reported a history of motion sickness in 50% of migraineurs versus only 20% of tension headache sufferers.[12] Motion sickness has been described as abdominal discomfort, dizziness, and headache occurring secondary to a neural mismatch between the visual system and the vestibular and/or proprioceptive systems. This mechanism is believed mediated at the level of the brainstem nuclei and the cerebellum. The connection between migraine and motion sickness tolerance was further delineated when it was shown that there was a statistically significant increase in photophobia, nausea, and duration of headache in migraine patients after optokinetic stimulation compared with normal controls.[13]

Visual-Vestibular Mismatch

The noxious visual stimuli inciting dizziness in these patients include reading; scrolling on a computer screen; watching action footage on television or in the movies; seeing highly patterned objects, such as quilts or checkerboard designs; being in busy situations, such as a store; and switching gaze back and forth between a computer monitor and written material. This so-called supermarket syndrome was introduced in 1975[14] to describe a subset of patients with Meniere syndrome whose primary complaints were visual in nature. A later compilation of case reports highlighted the challenge of dizzy patients whose complaints were primarily nonrotational dizziness, blurred and double vision, and visual motion hypersensitivity and for whom there seemed no clear diagnosis and no treatment.[15] Visual motion triggering or exacerbating dizziness has also been termed space and motion discomfort, visuo-vestibular mismatch, visual vertigo syndrome, and motorist disorientation syndrome.[16,17] On vestibular testing, these patients may have negative results or may demonstrate chronic abnormalities. Although in some of these patients, incorporating visual desensitization to vestibular rehabilitation has demonstrated benefits in both subjective symptoms and postural stability, many others cannot tolerate or find benefit from vestibular rehabilitation.[18]

Diagnostic Criteria for MAV

The currently accepted criteria[9] for definite MAV include current or prior history of migraine with episodic vertigo accompanied by headache, photophobia, phonophobia, and visual or other auras. The criteria for probable MAV include current or prior history of migraine, migrainous symptoms during vertigo, migraine precipitants of vertigo more than 50% of the time (including food triggers, sleep irregularities, or hormonal change), and greater than 50% response to migraine medications.

DIAGNOSIS

A detailed and thorough history helps distinguish between vestibular and nonvestibular headache.[19] Of particular importance in these individuals is a history of visually triggered vertigo and/or migraine. Much of what is known about this is derived from understanding of traumatic brain injury.[20] Questions that should be asked specifically include the following: Are you able to be in a supermarket aisle without feeling dizzy? Are you able to watch handheld camera footage or 3-D movies? Do you feel worse when scrolling on a computer or reading for periods of time or switching between printed materials and a computer monitor? Do you have difficulty in highly patterned or visually stimulating circumstances? A personal or family history of migraine headaches or Meniere syndrome or dizziness/vertigo in childhood is helpful in determining MAV. Diagnostic criteria for definite and probable MAV are detailed previously.

Physical examination related to MAV and visual-vestibular dysfunction is a complete ear-nose-throat-head-and-neck examination and additional tests. A user-friendly tool is the 10-minute examination of the dizzy patient.[21] It includes the following:

1. Spontaneous nystagmus
2. Gaze nystagmus
3. Smooth pursuit
4. Saccades
5. Fixation suppression
6. Head thrust
7. Post-headshake nystagmus
8. Dynamic visual acuity
9. Dix-Hallpike test
10. Static positional nystagmus evaluation
11. Limb coordination
12. Romberg stance
13. Gait observation
14. Specialized tests

Tests with which otolaryngologists are generally less familiar but that have a high rate of abnormality in MAV or visual-vestibular mismatch are screening tests of neuro-optometric function. These include the following:

1. Vergence oculomotor motility, looking for disjunctive changes of eye position in depth (ie, along the Z axis), including convergence, divergence, supravergence, and infravergence (Fig. 1A)
2. Versional ocular motility, examining conjunctive eye movements in a 2-D plane (ie, the X-Y plane), including fixation, saccades, and smooth pursuit (Fig. 1B)
3. Accommodation: which is the ability to change focus while retaining the clarity of vision while looking from near to far and back again, due to a change in the crystalline lens of the eye (Fig. 1)

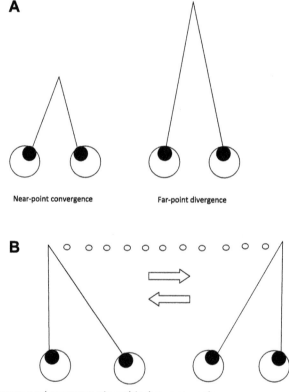

Fig. 1. (A) Vergence oculomotor testing: this shows normal eye convergence and divergence to near and far testing. Normal point of maximal convergence is 8–10 cm from the nose, and increases somewhat with age.* Although not shown here, testing should also be done for supravergence – where one eye rotates upward while the other remains still, and infravergence – where one eye rotates downward while the other remains still.** (B) Version testing: fixation, saccades, and smooth pursuit. (* Data from Fite JD, Walker HK. Clinical Methods: The History, Physical and Laboratory Examinations, 3rd Edition. Chapter 60 – Cranial Nerves III, IV, and VI: The Oculomotor, Trochlear, and Abducens Nerves. Part 1: Conjugate Gaze. Walker HK, Hall WD, Hurst JW, editors. Boston: Butterworths; 1990. ** Data from Grosvenor TP. Chapter 11: The Binocular Visual Examination. Grosvenor T. Primary Care Optometry. Elsevier Health Sciences, 2007.)

These tests can be done in an otolaryngologist's office; referral for neuro-optometric or neuro-ophthalmologic evaluation should be done in cases of abnormal findings. An even simpler test of oculomotor contribution to headache/vertigo is waving the examiner's hand close to a patient's face. A patient with visual-vestibular dysfunction pulls away or closes eyes immediately at the noxious stimulus.

Otovestibular testing, which may be ordered depending on the findings of the examination, include audiogram, video-electronystagmography, electrocochleography, and VEMP testing. Abnormal vestibular function is seen between episodes in both vertiginous and nonvertiginous migraine, and it is seen twice as often in vertiginous migraine patients than in nonvertiginous migraineurs (70% vs 34%).[22] There is no predilection for either central or peripheral vestibular abnormalities in either group. This implies that subclinical vestibular dysfunction may be a feature of migraine in general. When comparing patients with Meniere syndrome to those with migrainoid vertigo, vestibular test abnormalities are seen in 84% and 66%, respectively.[23] With decreasing incidence, headshake nystagmus, vibration-induced nystagmus, and caloric testing showed abnormalities in both groups.

Of another 30 patients with definitive MAV, the half with migrainous vertigo and vestibular abnormalities performed poorly in stabilometric examinations and seemed to rely more on visual cues in balance control than the half with migrainous vertigo but without vestibular abnormalities.[24] Migraneurs, even without definitive MAV, have defective oculomotor function, mostly of vestibulocerebellar origin.[25] This may explain the poorer performance of patients with MAV with additional oculomotor abnormalities overall.

Imaging for headache is described in detail elsewhere in this issue. Nonspecific white matter changes are frequently reported on brain MRI scan in migraine. If there is a unilateral audiovestibular finding on other testing, MRI should be ordered to rule out retrocochlear (internal auditory canal/brainstem) pathology. If there is a unilateral weak response on VEMP, thin-cut targeted CT images of the temporal bone are evaluated to look for superior semicircular canal dehiscence (SSCD), also called Minor's syndrome.

TREATMENT

When a diagnosis of MAV is made, treatment should first be directed at treating and/or prophylaxing the migraine headache component. This can be done with dietary modification as well as medications. Such treatment is beneficial in approximately three-quarters of patients with MAV.[26] Meniere-type findings are amenable to treatment that includes sodium and caffeine restriction, avoidance of dehydration, avoidance of nicotine, diuretics, and occasional use of short-term steroids. Long-term vestibular suppression is not recommended. Vestibular rehabilitation therapy is not beneficial in patients who do not have a fixed lesion, such as those with active Meniere syndrome or recurrent episodic MAV. This is particularly true in patients without stable ocular motor systems, because vestibular rehabilitation therapy relies on the fixed eye gaze for stability.

In patients with MAV and oculomotor abnormalities, addition of programmatic VT seems useful in recovery.[27] VT techniques use ocular motility exercises to train gradual visual sensitization,[28] seen in **Fig. 2**, and include the following exercises.

Exercise 1—Fist Passes

The patient is seated 6 to 8 feet from an empty wall with arms outstretched and hands in a fist. The outstretched fist is then slowly passed 40° to the left of center and then to

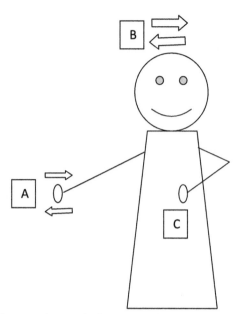

Fig. 2. Vision Rehabilitation Therapy (VT) exercises: (A) Fist passes, (B) Slow head rotations and (C) Convergence jumps.

40° right of center and then back to the midline, while being pursued visually without moving the head. This equals 1 repetition. Exercises are initiated at 10 repetitions per day and slowly increased to 12 to 15 repetitions by week 4. Starting at two weeks, blank colored self-adhesive (Post-it® type) notes are added to the wall 2 feet apart at eye level to slowly increase visual complexity of the background environment. Two more blank notes are added to the wall in each subsequent week until 6 blank notes are tolerated in the background. After 5 weeks of treatment, complexity is increased by altering position from seated to standing and, finally, marching in place as tolerated.

Exercise 2—Slow Head Rotations

The patient is seated 6 to 8 feet from an empty wall with arms outstretched and hands in a fist. The head is slowly turned 25° to 30° to the left of the midline target, then 25° to 30° to the right, and then back to the midline target. This equals 1 repetition. Exercises are initiated at 10 repetitions per day and slowly increased to 12 to 15 repetitions by week 4. Starting at 2 weeks, blank notes are added to the wall, as described previously, until 6 notes are tolerated in the background. Again, after 5 weeks of treatment, complexity is increased by altering position from seated to standing and, finally, marching in place as tolerated.

Exercise 3—Convergence Jumps

The patient is seated 6 to 8 feet from an empty wall. The right arm is fully outstretched and the thumb is pointed toward the ceiling. The left arm is outstretched and bent 90° at the elbow with the thumb pointed toward the ceiling. The patient then focuses on the left thumb for 3 seconds before transferring gaze to right thumb for 3 seconds. Gaze is then returned to the left thumb for 3 additional seconds. This equals 1 repetition.

Exercises are maintained at 5 repetitions per day throughout the course of therapy. Starting at 2 weeks, blank notes are added to the wall, as detailed previously, to a maximum of 6 notes. Similarly, after 5 weeks of treatment, complexity is increased by altering position from seated to standing and, finally, marching in place as tolerated.

LONG-TERM PROGNOSIS

Long-term evaluation of patients with definite MAV reveals persistence, and sometimes worsening of, the otologic portion of their syndrome. Nine years after MAV diagnosis, 61 patients were evaluated[29]:

- 87% Had recurrent vertigo at follow-up.
- Frequency of vertigo was reduced in 56%, increased in 29%, and unchanged in 16%.
- Impact of vertigo was severe in 21%, moderate in 43%, and mild in 36%.
- 18% Reported mild persistent unsteadiness.
- Concomitant cochlear symptoms with vertigo had increased from 15% initially to 49%.
- Eleven patients (18%) had developed mild bilateral sensorineural hearing loss, which also involved the low-frequency range.

In that same study, eye findings were more heterogeneous. Interepisode ocular motor abnormalities increased from 16% initially to 41% of patients at follow-up. Only 1 of 9 patients with ocular motor abnormalities at initial presentation, however, showed similar findings on follow-up.

Patient Story: Dizziness and Imbalance

A 31-year-old woman presented with severe imbalance while driving for slightly more than 1 year, progressing to inability to drive for the past 8 months, wherein she thought that she and the car would topple to the opposite side away from a curve in the road, and she was unable to change lanes to the left on a highway. She experienced dizziness and tiredness after using the computer at work and felt dizzy in narrow alleys. Audiovestibular testing revealed normal hearing, electrocochleography, auditory brainstem response, and VEMPs. Video-electronystagmography demonstrated right-beating nystagmus that suppressed with vision. A brain MRI scan demonstrated white matter changes consistent with migraine. Initial migraine treatment included acetazolamide, with slight benefit. Over time, migraine headaches manifested themselves with changing intensity. Neuro-optometric evaluation revealed convergence insufficiency, and home-based VT was instituted. Within 3 weeks, she was able to resume many of her driving duties and no longer became tired after computer use at work. The more complicated VT exercises, however, seemed to trigger the patient's migraines. She was then begun on oral topiramate, which successfully ameliorated her migraines. She continued with VT and subsequently returned to full driving and working capabilities.

SUMMARY

Migraine-associated dizziness is an evolving clinical entity. Recognition of the historical and physical examination features among these patients is necessary guide treatment. Aggressive dietary and medication management of the migraine is effective in 70% of patients. Ocular dysmotility in migraineurs may induce a chronic neuronal mismatch between the visual and vestibular systems that manifests as dizziness and disequilibrium. This subset of MAV patients is often refractory to current standard treatment modalities and is frequently dismissed as having psychogenic issues. Addition of vision treatment to address the underlying oculomotor dysfunction can be beneficial in these individuals. Long-term follow-up is important, because their otologic abnormalities, including dizziness, vertigo, and hearing loss, may manifest only later in the clinical course.

ACKNOWLEDGMENTS

My sincere gratitude to Dr Neera Kapoor, OD, MS, FAOO, Director, R Greenwald Center, State University of New York, State University Optometric Center, for educating me about the intersection of our specialties and for teaching me how to offer better treatment to patients.

REFERENCES

1. Osler W. Osler's "A Way of Life" and other addresses, with commentary and annotations. Durham (NC), London: Duke University Press; 2001.
2. Ravishankar K. The art of history-taking in a headache patient. Ann Indian Acad Neurol 2012;15(Suppl 1):S7–14.
3. Davies MB. How do I diagnose headache? J Roy Coll Phys Edinb 2006;36: 336–42.
4. Kanagalingam J, Hajioff D, Bennett S. Vertigo. BMJ 2005;330:523.
5. Labuguen RH. Initial evaluation of vertigo. Am Fam Physician 2006;73(2):244–51.
6. Koenigsberger MR, Chandrasekhar SS. El nino con mareos. Rev Neurol 1995; 23(Suppl 3):S410–7.
7. Szirmai A. Vestibular disorders in childhood and adolescents. Eur Arch Otorhinolaryngol 2010;267(11):1801–4.
8. Neuhauser H, Leopold M, von Brevern M, et al. The interrelations of migraine, vertigo, and migranous vertigo. Neurology 2001;56(4):436–41.
9. Neuhauser H, Lempert T. Vertigo and dizziness related to migraine: a diagnostic challenge. Cephalalgia 2004;24:83–91.
10. Headache classification committee of the international headache society. The international classification of headache disorders, 2nd edition. Cephalalgia 2004; 24(Suppl 1):1–160.
11. Furman JM, Sparto PJ, Soso M, et al. Vestibular function in migraine-related dizziness: a pilot study. J Vestib Res 2005;15:327–32.
12. Kayan A, Hood JD. Neuro-otologic manifestations of migraine. Brain 1984; 107(Pt 4):1123–42.
13. Drummond PD. Motion sickness and migraine: optokinetic stimulation increases scalp tenderness, pain sensitivity in fingertips and photophobia. Cephalalgia 2002;22:117–24.
14. McCabe BF. Diseases of the end organ and vestibular nerve. In: Naunton RF, editor. The vestibular system. New York: Academic Press; 1975. p. 299–302.
15. Hoffman RA, Brookler KH. Underrated neurotologic symptoms. Laryngoscope 1978;88(7 Pt 1):1127–38.
16. Ciuffreda KJ. Visual vertigo syndrome: clinical demonstration and diagnostic tool. Clin Eye Vis Care 1999;11:41–2.
17. Guerraz M, Yardley I, Bertholon P, et al. Visual vertigo: symptom assessment, spatial orientation and postural control. Brain 2001;124(Pt 8):1646–56.
18. Pavlou M, Lingeswaran A, Davies RA, et al. Simulator based rehabilitation in refractory dizziness. J Neurol 2004;251:983–95.
19. Zhao JG, Piccirillo JF, Spitznagel EL Jr, et al. Predictive capability of historical data for diagnosis of dizziness. Otol Neurotol 2011;32(2):284–90.
20. Kapoor N, Ciuffreda KJ. Vision disturbances following traumatic brain injury. Curr Treat Options Neurol 2002;4:271–80.

21. Goebel JA. The ten-minute examination of the dizzy patient. Semin Neurol 2001; 21(4):391–8.
22. Boldingh MI, Ljøstad U, Mygland A, et al. Comparison of interictal vestibular function in vestibular migraine vs migraine without vertigo. Headache 2013;53(7): 1123–33.
23. Shin JE, Kim CH, Park HJ. Vestibular abnormality in patients with Meniere's disease and migrainous vertigo. Acta Otolaryngol 2013;133(2):154–8.
24. Teggi R, Colombo B, Bernasconi L, et al. Migrainous vertigo: results of caloric testing and stabilometric findings. Headache 2009;49(3):435–44.
25. Harno H, Hirvonen T, Kaunisto MA, et al. Subclinical vestibulocerebellar dysfunction in migraine with and without aura. Neurology 2003;61(12):1748–52.
26. Fotuhi M, Glaun B, Quan SY, et al. Vestibular migraine: a critical review of treatment trials. J Neurol 2009;256(5):711–6.
27. Cohen AH, Rein LD. The effect of head trauma on the visual system: the doctor of optometry as a member of the rehabilitation team. J Am Optom Assoc 1992; 63(8):530–6.
28. Ciuffreda KJ, Han Y, Kapoor N, et al. Oculomotor rehabilitation for reading in acquired brain injury. NeuroRehabilitation 2006;21(1):9–21.
29. Radtke A, von Brevern M, Neuhauser H, et al. Vestibular migraine: long-term follow-up of clinical symptoms and vestibulo-cochlear findings. Neurology 2012;79(15):1607–14.

The Neurosurgical Treatment of Neuropathic Facial Pain

Jeffrey A. Brown, MD

KEYWORDS

- Trigeminal neuralgia • Microvascular decompression • Neuropathic facial pain
- Radiosurgery • Balloon compression • Atypical facial pain

KEY POINTS

- When facial pain persists or develops after rhinologic surgery and there is no apparent rhinologic cause, a neuropathic cause should be considered, and the next level of investigation should be of the trigeminal nerve root.
- A neuropathic origin for facial pain should be considered when evaluating a patient for rhinologic surgery because of complaints of facial pain.
- Neuropathic facial pain is caused by vascular compression of the trigeminal nerve in the prepontine cistern and is characterized by an intermittent prickling or stabbing component or a constant burning, searing pain.
- Medical treatment consists of anticonvulsant medication.
- Neurosurgical treatment may require microvascular decompression of the trigeminal nerve.

CASE HISTORY

A 53-year-old woman had undergone sinus surgery for repeated episodes of sinusitis. She had persistent left maxillary sinus pain and tenderness aggravated by cool air touching her face. A dentist performed a root canal. It aggravated her pain and she had an extraction. Her pain became searing in quality and she said that it felt like a poker in her face. Pregabalin, an anticonvulsant used to treat pain of neuropathic origin, helped, but she became allergic to it.

Her magnetic resonance imaging (MRI) scan showed a vascular association in the root entry zone of the left trigeminal nerve and a possible second site of compression of the trigeminal nerve at the entrance to the Meckel cave (**Fig. 1A**).

She underwent a microvascular decompression of the trigeminal nerve. The superior cerebellar artery tented up the nerve and was in contact with it throughout its

The author reports no actual or potential conflict of interest, including employment, consultancies, stock ownership, patent applications/registrations/grants, or other funding.
Neurological Surgery, PC, 600 Northern Boulevard #118, Great Neck, NY 11021, USA
E-mail address: jbrown@nspc.com

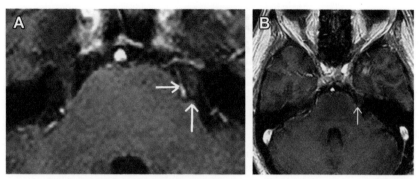

Fig. 1. (*A*) Magnetic resonance image through the trigeminal nerve at the pontine level. Vertical arrow points to the left trigeminal nerve root. Horizontal arrow points to the superior cerebellar artery, which contacts the nerve root throughout its cisternal course. (*B*) Magnetic resonance image showing the left trigeminal nerve (*arrow*) after decompression by mobilization of the superior cerebellar artery.

prepontine cisternal segment. The arterial loop was mobilized and separated from the nerve with felt (see **Fig. 1**B).

By 2 months after surgery her score on the McGill Pain Questionnaire had decreased to 9 from her preoperative score of 68. There was some residual burning sensation, whereas the preoperative pain was described as searing.

INTRODUCTION
Why Sinus Surgery for Pain Fails to Relieve that Pain, and Why Seemingly Successful Rhinologic Surgery Leads to Chronic Facial/Head Pain

This article answers these questions and reviews the definition, etiology and evaluation, and medical and surgical treatment of neuropathic facial pain.

Important Points

When facial pain persists or develops after rhinologic surgery and there is no apparent rhinologic cause, a neuropathic cause should be considered and the next level of investigation should be of the trigeminal nerve root. A neuropathic origin for facial pain should also be considered when evaluating a patient for possible rhinologic surgery because of complaints of facial pain.

Definitions

There are 2 classes of facial pain: nociceptive and neuropathic.

Nociceptive pain arises from a noxious stimulus that causes damage to non-neural tissue. An irritating stimulus activates nociceptive neurons of the central or peripheral somatosensory system that encode, transduce, and transmit it to the spinal cord and brain.[1]

Nociceptive facial pain is most commonly caused by trauma, tumor, or infection.

Medical treatment of nociceptive pain focuses on the use of antibiotics, antiinflammatory medication, and opioids. Antiinflammatory effects are peripheral. Opioid effects are central.

Neuropathic pain is a clinical entity caused by injury to the peripheral or central somatosensory nervous system. Neuropathic pain is characterized by the presence of hyperpathia, hyperalgesia, allodynia, and hypoalgesia.

Hyperalgesia or hypoalgesia means increased or decreased pain from a stimulus that normally causes pain. Allodynia means that a stimulus that normally is not painful causes pain.

Dysesthesias are unpleasant, abnormal sensations that may be spontaneous or provoked. Dysesthesias may be constant or intermittent. When intermittent, they are described in spatial terms as (in order of increasing severity) jumping, flashing, or shooting; in punctate terms (in increasing severity) they are pricking, boring, drilling, stabbing, or lancinating; in incisive terms (in increasing severity) they are sharp, cutting, or lacerating.[2] More severe spatial, punctate, or incisive pain tends to be intermittent. The International Association of Pain considers a paresthesia to be an abnormal sensation that is not unpleasant.[1] For the purposes of this article, paresthesias are intermittent electrical sensations that have spatial or incisive components to them. As such, patients describe them as stabbing, lancinating, sharp, cutting, or lacerating.

Facial neuropathic pain may have a predominance of paresthesias or dysesthesias.

Descriptors of dysesthesias in the McGill Pain Questionnaire include categories of thermal pain such as the terms hot, burning, scalding, and searing.[2] Thermal dysesthesias tend to be constant.

The presence of constant dysesthesias is important in determining the nature of the neurosurgical treatment. Current neurosurgical treatment options include ablation, decompression, or modulation.

Ablation is a means of injuring the trigeminal system. The most common neurosurgical target for injury to the trigeminal system is the trigeminal nerve root, which is found within the subarachnoid space ventral to the pons, between the trigeminal ganglion and the pons. Techniques for nerve root injury (in order of historical development) include (1) thermal injury (radiofrequency rhizotomy), (2) chemical (glycerol rhizotomy),[3] (3) mechanical (balloon compression),[4] (4) radiosurgery (fixed cobalt source radiation–based [Gamma Knife] and linear accelerator–based [robotic-CyberKnife or multileaf collimator; Novalis]).[5–7]

Microvascular decompression consists of surgical manipulation of an artery or vein away from the trigeminal nerve root surface.[8]

Neuromodulation techniques include peripheral trigeminal stimulation or central, motor cortex stimulation.[9]

The medical treatment of neuropathic pain primarily consists of oral anticonvulsant medications, such as carbamazepine or gabapentin. The medical treatment of dysesthesias and paresthesias is similar. Anticonvulsant drugs slow electrical conductivity in the nervous system, which stops seizures. It also reduces the electrical input to the short circuit in the trigeminal system that occurs because of the vascular compression and causes the pain. This medication effect also slows cognition and coordination.[10–13]

Facial pain may be solely nociceptive, neuropathic, or it may be mixed.

Neuropathic pain may derive from vascular compression of the trigeminal nerve root; surgical or traumatic injury to the trigeminal root, ganglion, or peripheral branches; tumor; stroke; or demyelinating disease.

Evaluation of the Patient with Facial Pain

The first goal of such an evaluation is to learn whether the patient's pain is nociceptive, neuropathic, or a mixture. It is helpful to have the patient complete a long-form McGill Pain Questionnaire to do this. The use of descriptives in the categories of spatial, punctate, incisive, or thermal suggests a neuropathic component to the pain. Pain that is burning, searing, stabbing, or lancinating is neuropathic. Pain that is tender, aching, gnawing, throbbing, or dull is nociceptive.

A neurologic examination should focus on motor and sensory testing of the trigeminal system. Temperature, light touch, and pinprick (pain) sensation should be tested in all 3 trigeminal divisions. There may be hypoesthesia or hyperesthesia. The corneal reflex may be depressed or absent.

Jaw opening tests the pterygoid muscles. The motor root of the trigeminal nerve via the mandibular branch mediates pterygoid muscle function. If there is unilateral weakness, the jaw deviates to the ipsilateral side when opened. There may be eustachian tube dysfunction. The tensor veli palatini and tensor tympani muscles are innervated by the motor mandibular nerve and participate in eustachian tube function. Dysfunction occurs if there is compression of the nerve by a tumor, such as a trigeminal schwannoma.

If there is a tumor, or there has been a stroke, other cranial nerves may be affected. This condition may involve the vestibular system, extraocular movement, facial muscle function, or innervation of the posterior tongue and pharynx.

Imaging

MRI of the trigeminal nerve is not a component of a standard MRI study. A technique that shows the relationship between arteries, veins, and the trigeminal nerve in thin-cut sequences is required. On a Siemens MRI system it is called a constructive interference with steady state (CISS) gradient-echo sequence.[14] On a General Electric MRI system it is called a fast imaging employing steady state acquisition cycled phases (FIESTA) technique.[15] Such sequences provide excellent contrast between cerebrospinal fluid in the prepontine cisternal space, the trigeminal nerve, and other blood vessels.

Diagnosis

When a rhinologic or odontologic cause of chronic facial pain cannot be determined, a neuropathic cause should be investigated. Begin with the hypothesis that peripheral trigeminal injury/irritation at the time of facial surgery can initiate a predisposition to a short circuit in the trigeminal system. That predisposition is a result of vascular compression of the prepontine cisternal segment of the trigeminal nerve. The compression can be arterial or venous, or both. The prognosis differs according to the nature of the compression. Such compression causes altered histopathology and electrophysiology of myelinated trigeminal fibers.

Intraoperative biopsies have been done of the affected trigeminal root beneath the site of compression during surgery. They show zones of demyelination and dysmyelination, juxtaposition of denuded axons, axon loss and degeneration, and collagen deposition. Ultrastructural evaluation revealed dysmyelination and axons devoid of myelin adjacent to each other. This finding is consistent with neurophysiologic hypotheses of pain production by ectopic discharges, ephaptic transmission between axons without myelin, and crossed afterdischarge.[16]

Microvascular Decompression

In one of the largest series of patients with neuropathic facial pain, 1185 patients were evaluated for at least 1 year after microvascular decompression (MVD).[8,17] Ten years after their surgery, 70% of the patients were free of pain without medication. Pain recurred in one-third of the patients and 11% required a second operation for the recurrence. Most recurrences were in the first 2 years. Pain for more than 8 years before surgery, findings of venous compression, and delayed pain relief after surgery were significant factors for pain recurrence. Stroke, hearing loss, or death occurred in less than 1% of patients.

If pain is constant, results of MVD surgery are not as beneficial as they are when there is intermittent, stabbing pain. In a series of 135 patients who had an MVD and were evaluated for a median period of 3 years, pain relief was better (81%) if the pain was intermittent, but only 77% if the pain had been constant.[18]

There is no published series of results of MVD in patients who underwent dental or sinus surgery before the onset of neuropathic pain.

The intermittent severe paresthesias of classic trigeminal neuralgia are surgically treated by MVD or an ablative procedure.[19] The hypothesis is that proximal demyelinating trigeminal nerve injury reduces the electrical input to the presumed short circuit in the nerve. This process turns off the switch that triggers the electrical surge of the short circuit. Mild to moderate sensory loss is better tolerated than the paresthesias of trigeminal neuralgia.

Ablative Procedures

Radiofrequency thermal rhizotomy is a percutaneous treatment of trigeminal neuralgia done by selectively heating the involved trigeminal nerve root and reevaluating the wakened patient until a goal of mild to moderate hypoesthesia is attained. Selective injury is possible because of the anatomic organization of the trigeminal nerve root. Mandibular fibers are ventral and ophthalmic fibers are dorsal in the root, which is located in the prepontine cistern. Selectivity is achieved by using a percutaneously inserted electrode with a curved tip. A series of timed lesions are made and the patients are repeatedly reexamined.[19] Lower levels of heat selectively injure unmyelinated pain fibers. However, injury sufficient to cause hypoesthesia is not fiber specific.

Balloon compression creates an injury specific to a fiber type. Compression selectively injures the large myelinated fibers that mediate light touch. These fibers conduct the electrical trigger to the paresthesias of the neuralgic pain. Nerve root compression is done for 1 minute to a pressure of 1.5 atm, which creates a demyelinating injury in the preganglionic root of the trigeminal nerve. It also eliminates the trigger to the trigeminal paresthesias of the short circuit in the nerve.

Glycerol also creates a chemical demyelination of the nerve. It can be done selectively by increasing the volume of the chemical injected into the trigeminal cistern containing the ganglion. Higher volumes are needed to reach the maxillary and ophthalmic divisions.[20]

Neuromodulation

Dental or rhinologic procedures may promote the onset of neuropathic pain. The chronic facial pain is then not a consequence of any peripheral nerve injury that may have occurred during the surgery because the cause of the pain is central, not peripheral.

When the facial pain is constant and burning, ablative operations may worsen the pain by further injuring the trigeminal nerve.[21] Surgical options for constant, burning facial pain are MVD or neuromodulation. These procedures are designed to preserve trigeminal function.

Options for neuromodulation include peripheral trigeminal stimulation and motor cortex stimulation.

Contralateral epidural motor cortex stimulation is postulated to be effective for constant neuropathic facial pain by inhibiting the thalamic hyperactivity that occurs after injury to facial sensory fiber input.[9] Subthreshold stimulation of the facial motor cortex leads to a 50% to 75% reduction in constant burning facial pain and comparable reduction in pain medication requirements.[22]

Subcutaneous peripheral trigeminal branch stimulation for constant neuropathic face has more recently been used. Electrodes may be percutaneously positioned over the infraorbital, supraorbital, preauricular, or nasolabial trigeminal branches to treat medically intractable pain in the comparable facial regions.

Radiosurgery

Focused beam injury of the trigeminal nerve root is not division selective and pain relief is delayed for a period of weeks until the radiation injury becomes effective. Gamma knife radiosurgery uses a fixed source of cobalt radiation that delivers a 4-mm collimated beam 2 to 4 mm anterior to the junction of the trigeminal nerve and the pons.[5] The target is centered on the targeting beam by fixing the patient's head in a stereotactic frame that is secured to the skull as an outpatient procedure. With Cyber-Knife radiosurgery, a robotic arm homogeneously and sequentially delivers approximately 100 collimated beams to a 6-mm length of the trigeminal nerve. Skull radiographs repeatedly performed at intervals during the delivery are fused with preoperative computed tomography images. This fusion allows compensations to be made in the targeting because of minor head movement. In this way a fixed frame is not required.[23]

All ablative procedures have an inherent likelihood of pain recurrence higher than that seen with MVD. Ablation of the trigeminal nerve is primarily demyelinating. Because myelin regeneration does occur, the sensory loss after injury may gradually resolve, leading to recurrence of pain.[24]

The knowledge base required to achieve optimal diagnosis and treatment of facial pain encompasses the knowledge and expertise of rhinologic, plastic, oral-maxillary, and neurologic surgeons. As such, facial pain can remain a diagnostic dilemma to the physician/surgeon who is less familiar with the focus of these other specialties and subspecialties. This article outlines the principles that are important to understanding the nature of chronic facial pain and reviews important aspects of the neurosurgical treatment of neuropathic facial pain.

REFERENCES

1. Merskey H. The taxonomy of pain. Med Clin North Am 2007;91(1):13–20, vii.
2. Melzack R. The McGill Pain Questionnaire: major properties and scoring methods. Pain 1975;1(3):277–99.
3. Kouzounias K, Lind G, Schechtmann G, et al. Comparison of percutaneous balloon compression and glycerol rhizotomy for the treatment of trigeminal neuralgia. J Neurosurg 2010;113(3):486–92.
4. Brown JA. Percutaneous balloon compression for trigeminal neuralgia. Clin Neurosurg 2009;56:73–8.
5. Kondziolka D, Zorro O, Lobato-Polo J, et al. Gamma knife stereotactic radiosurgery for idiopathic trigeminal neuralgia. J Neurosurg 2010;112(4):758–65.
6. Fariselli L, Marras C, De Santis M, et al. CyberKnife radiosurgery as a first treatment for idiopathic trigeminal neuralgia. Neurosurgery 2009;64(Suppl 2): A96–101.
7. Zahra H, Teh BS, Paulino AC, et al. Stereotactic radiosurgery for trigeminal neuralgia utilizing the BrainLAB Novalis system. Technol Cancer Res Treat 2009;8(6): 407–12.
8. Barker FG 2nd, Jannetta PJ, Bissonette DJ, et al. The long-term outcome of microvascular decompression for trigeminal neuralgia. N Engl J Med 1996; 334(17):1077–83.

9. Brown JA, Pilitsis JG. Motor cortex stimulation for central and neuropathic facial pain: a prospective study of 10 patients and observations of enhanced sensory and motor function during stimulation. Neurosurgery 2005;56(2):290–7 [discussion: 290–7].

10. Delcker A, Wilhelm H, Timmann D, et al. Side effects from increased doses of carbamazepine on neuropsychological and posturographic parameters of humans. Eur Neuropsychopharmacol 1997;7(3):213–8.

11. Martin R, Meador K, Turrentine L, et al. Comparative cognitive effects of carbamazepine and gabapentin in healthy senior adults. Epilepsia 2001;42(6):764–71.

12. Salinsky MC, Binder LM, Oken BS, et al. Effects of gabapentin and carbamazepine on the EEG and cognition in healthy volunteers. Epilepsia 2002;43(5): 482–90.

13. Kaussner Y, Kenntner-Mabiala R, Hoffmann S, et al. Effects of oxcarbazepine and carbamazepine on driving ability: a double-blind, randomized crossover trial with healthy volunteers. Psychopharmacology 2010;210(1):53–63.

14. Yousry I, Moriggl B, Schmid UD, et al. Trigeminal ganglion and its divisions: detailed anatomic MR imaging with contrast-enhanced 3D constructive interference in the steady state sequences. AJNR Am J Neuroradiol 2005;26(5): 1128–35.

15. Wang TJ, Brisman R, Lu ZF, et al. Image registration strategy of T(1)-weighted and FIESTA MRI sequences in trigeminal neuralgia Gamma knife radiosurgery. Stereotact Funct Neurosurg 2010;88(4):239–45.

16. Rappaport ZH, Govrin-Lippmann R, Devor M. An electron-microscopic analysis of biopsy samples of the trigeminal root taken during microvascular decompressive surgery. Stereotact Funct Neurosurg 1997;68(1–4 Pt 1):182–6.

17. Tyler-Kabara EC, Kassam AB, Horowitz MH, et al. Predictors of outcome in surgically managed patients with typical and atypical trigeminal neuralgia: comparison of results following microvascular decompression. J Neurosurg 2002;96(3): 527–31.

18. Sandell T, Eide PK. Effect of microvascular decompression in trigeminal neuralgia patients with or without constant pain. Neurosurgery 2008;63(1):93–9 [discussion: 99–100].

19. Taha JM, Tew JM Jr, Buncher CR. A prospective 15-year follow up of 154 consecutive patients with trigeminal neuralgia treated by percutaneous stereotactic radiofrequency thermal rhizotomy. J Neurosurg 1995;83(6):989–93.

20. Lunsford LD. Treatment of tic douloureux by percutaneous retrogasserian glycerol injection. JAMA 1982;248(4):449–53.

21. Brown JA. Motor cortex stimulation. Neurosurg Focus 2001;11(3):E5.

22. Fontaine D, Hamani C, Lozano A. Efficacy and safety of motor cortex stimulation for chronic neuropathic pain: critical review of the literature. J Neurosurg 2009; 110(2):251–6.

23. Borchers JD 3rd, Yang HJ, Sakamoto GT, et al. Cyberknife stereotactic radiosurgical rhizotomy for trigeminal neuralgia: anatomic and morphological considerations. Neurosurgery 2009;64(Suppl 2):A91–5.

24. Lopez BC, Hamlyn PJ, Zakrzewska JM. Systematic review of ablative neurosurgical techniques for the treatment of trigeminal neuralgia. Neurosurgery 2004; 54(4):973–82 [discussion: 982–3].

Index

Note: Page numbers of article titles are in **boldface** type.

Otolaryngol Clin N Am 47 (2014) 351–357
http://dx.doi.org/10.1016/S0030-6665(14)00009-7
0030-6665/14/$ – see front matter © 2014 Elsevier Inc. All rights reserved.

oto.theclinics.com

Moving?

Make sure your subscription moves with you!

To notify us of your new address, find your **Clinics Account Number** (located on your mailing label above your name), and contact customer service at:

Email: journalscustomerservice-usa@elsevier.com

800-654-2452 (subscribers in the U.S. & Canada)
314-447-8871 (subscribers outside of the U.S. & Canada)

Fax number: 314-447-8029

Elsevier Health Sciences Division
Subscription Customer Service
3251 Riverport Lane
Maryland Heights, MO 63043

*To ensure uninterrupted delivery of your subscription, please notify us at least 4 weeks in advance of move.

ELSEVIER

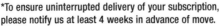

Printed and bound by CPI Group (UK) Ltd, Croydon, CR0 4YY

03/10/2024

01040497-0020